Fine Black Lines

Reflections on Facing
Cancer, Fear and Loneliness

Lois Tschetter Hjelmstad

MULBERRY HILL PRESS

Denver, Colorado

Mulberry Hill Press
P. O. Box 425-B
Englewood, Colorado   80151-0425

Editorial assistance: Peggy Cole
Cover design: Bruce Holdeman (adapted from a drawing by Peggy Cole)
Inside illustrations: JoRoan Lazaro
Page design: Karen Martin

The following were originally published as indicated:
    "No Lifeguard on Duty" and "When She Is Four" in *Progenitor* 1993
    "War" in *The Echo* 1991
    "Snow Lady," by Jim and Peggy Cole, as a color photograph in *Progenitor* 1986; reprinted with permission of Jim and Peggy Cole.

Publisher's Cataloging in Publication
    (Prepared by Quality Books, Inc.)

Hjelmstad, Lois Tschetter
        Fine black lines : reflections on facing cancer, fear, and loneliness / Lois Tschetter Hjelmstad.
        p. cm.
        Includes index.
        Preassigned Library of Congress Catalog Card Number: 93-78394.
        ISBN 0-9637139-5-7
        1. Hjelmstad, Lois Tschetter. 2. Breast–Cancer–Patients–Biography.
    3. Chronic fatigue syndrome–Patients–Biography. I. Title.

    RC280.B8H54 1993   362.19'699449'0092
                                                    QBI93-913

Printed in the United States of America
Published October 1993
Second Printing, April 1994
Third Printing, February 1995
Fourth Printing, August 1996

To my parents,
Paul and Bertha Tschetter,
who gave me life

To my husband, Les,
who has made life worth living

To my children,
Karen, Bob, Keith and Russ,
and my grandchildren,
who extend my life

Table of Contents

Foreword

Breast cancer is a life experience that produces change in a woman's life that is often profound, sometimes subtle. Whatever a woman's response, it forcefully causes her to focus on issues of mortality, self-esteem, survival, sexuality and a number of other things that give substance and meaning to life.

Having the privilege of working so closely with breast cancer patients over the past five years has had an incredible impact on my own life. These women have taught me many things, but paramount in their teaching has been that to survive and find meaning in the experience one must find a healthy blend of realism and optimism. Lois's book does this in a way that few other writings do. She is so profoundly honest in examining her own experience that it leaves me with a sense of genuine appreciation that she invited me to come along and share her journey. Lois's writing is also permeated with a sense of hope. However, I find it not to be that superficial kind of hope that simply smiles and says everything is fine. It is that deep, abiding hope that one can play the hand that is dealt, although there are times and circumstances that make one question that.

I would highly recommended this book not only to women experiencing breast cancer or those facing chronic illness, but to anyone who is traversing life.

June 9, 1993　　　　　　　Jeanne Currey, R.N., M.N., C.S.
Psychiatric Clinical Nurse Specialist
Oncology Services

About the Author and the Book

The author has been married for 44 years. She and her husband have four grown children (a daughter and three sons) and ten grandchildren. She has taught piano, music theory and composition for 31 years.

She loves walking, traveling, entertaining family and friends, teaching and being involved with children, and thinking about the larger issues of life.

The book focuses on the past four years of her life. It contains excerpts from her journal, selected poems, and reflections.

Insets and bracketed comments in the journals were added for clarification during the writing of the book.

Acknowledgments

I would never have chosen to have breast cancer, and I am not sure how grateful I am for the reasons I came to write this book. But I am profoundly grateful for the relationships, encouragement and healing that have come to me in the process. Fine and generous people have turned up, often unexpectedly, wanting to help. Without their willingness to assist, this project would not have become a reality. I want to thank each of them from the bottom of my heart:

♦ Peggy Cole, Ph.D., for encouraging me to include more journal entries and the bracketed and inset explanations, for pressing me to write the reflections and be true to my experiences, and for hours of editing. Her sensitive questioning clarified ideas and elicited deeper levels of truthfulness. Her careful attention to detail and structure helped transform the manuscript.

♦ Karen Hjelmstad Martin for early brainstorming, for suggesting that I include journal entries and prose with the poetry, for helping me keep my perspective, and for insisting that I continue with the project when it seemed too daunting. Her technical skill in typesetting and layout were also invaluable.

The endless patience, love and dedication of these two women gave me the strength to go on.

♦ My family and friends for reading drafts of the manuscript and for their suggestions, criticism and support.

♦ Ann Keener (who died of cancer August 28, 1991) for opening her heart to me. Her gentle, gracious spirit has illuminated my life.

♦ The women of my breast cancer support group for providing me with a sounding board and insisting that I not soften the truth. I will always treasure their insights, good humor and courage. To protect their privacy, I have given them fictitious names.

L.H.

Fine Black Lines

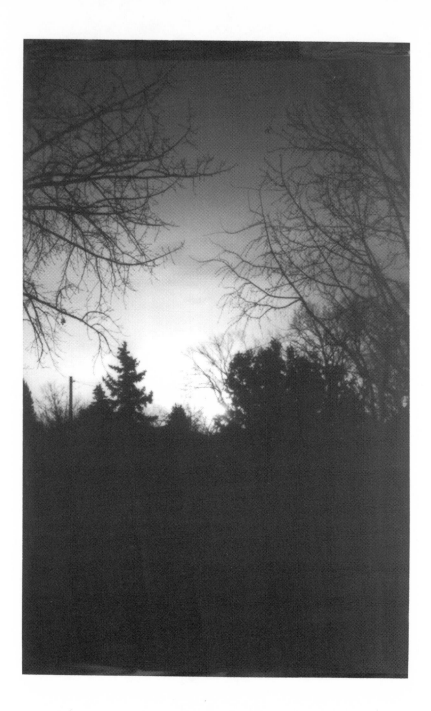

If I Could Stay Awake 'til Dawn

Parable

Once upon a time, there was a little girl who was terrified of The Dark. Sometimes she raced up the stairs, a monster nipping at her heels, and flew shrieking into the safety of her parents' bed.

When she was three, her mother let her play outdoors "alone." Her mother never worried because she knew the little girl's dog would be like a mother to her, going wherever she went. The dog always took care of her, nudging her out of harm's way.

One night Collie didn't come home for dinner. The little girl called and called into The Dark, her voice swept away on the wind. The emptiness echoed in her heart.

Later she learned that a neighbor had seen Collie near his sheep and shot her. It was the first time the little girl realized that things could be taken from her. Although she didn't understand exactly why, the thought terrified her. But she pretended to be a "big, brave girl."

The little girl wanted someone to take care of her, but she also wanted to "do it myself."

When she was four, her little brother was born and then she *had* to "do it myself." And she tried to protect her little brother from The Dark, too.

1

Then she found herself trying to take care of everyone. She didn't know what to do. After all, she *was* a very little girl. And she still wanted to be loved and rocked and held, especially when it was Dark. But everyone said, "You're a big girl now."

Her sister was born when she was eight, and the little girl tried to protect her whole family from The Dark.

When she was eleven, Pearl Harbor was bombed. It seemed to her as if Darkness enveloped the entire world. When Hiroshima was bombed, she felt sure the world would end before she could grow up.

In the threat of that shadow, she grew older, still pretending to be a big, brave girl.

She got married and became a mother. She had four children, and she rocked and held them, the way she had wanted to be held, trying to give them the hugs she had needed. But she always felt she was just playing house.

She was still a little girl, afraid of The Dark and sickness and accidents—and especially afraid of being left alone. She needed to be loved and rocked and held, especially when darkness fell.

After awhile she was able to tell her husband that she needed to be rocked and held, particularly when she was obstreperous. And he held her in his arms and rocked her. And sometimes it was almost enough.

But she was still a little girl and she was still afraid of The Final Dark—whether it fell first on him or first on her.

It was hard for her to play "grown-up." She was often scared. One day, however, she reflected on the grownup things she had somehow done.

She thought about the long years she had been alone at night with the children because her husband worked the graveyard shift.

She thought about the long night when her daughter was born nine weeks early and how she felt that if she could just stay awake until dawn she would somehow ensure the life of the three-pound baby.

She thought long and hard about how, 23 years later, she held that daughter in her arms—a widow before *she* was. She remembered how long that night had seemed and how she would have given anything—even her own dear husband—if the daughter could have awakened to a world that had not been shattered. She knew it would not help this time, but she stayed awake until dawn anyway.

She thought about her three sons and the long nights when she didn't know where they were or whether they would come home again—and how she had feared she could not keep them safe by staying awake until dawn.

She thought about the night she screamed and railed against God as her husband lay in a hospital, his body crushed in an accident. She wasn't sure tomorrow would come for him. If she could just stay awake until dawn....

She thought about the night, many years later, when her daughter's daughter was also born nine weeks too soon, and, overwhelmed by infection, they both almost died. She sat on a stiff chair in a hospital room until dawn, hoping against hope.

She thought about the first long night after she learned she had cancer. She ran, terrified, through the corridors of her mind, a monster nipping at her heels. When she whirled, she saw the monster duck behind a door. And then, knowing it was useless to stay awake until dawn, she closed her eyes and fell asleep.

And so it came to pass, that having glimpsed The Final Dark, the little girl found that she was stronger than she had realized.

She had lost her innocence and her belief that if she was a good girl everything would be okay. And she had learned

3

that Darkness is a gift—an opportunity to face mortality—however painful the process might be.

She was still afraid of The Dark. She still wanted to be rocked and held. The nights were sometimes very long.

But the little-girl-who-became-a-woman knew she would never be a little girl again....

And she had learned to treasure each new day as if it were the First Day.

January 1982
May 1993

Small Boy

(for Les)

I'd like to make the dreams come true
For that small boy who once was you...

I'd like to gently wipe the tears,
Kiss all the hurts and calm the fears...

I'd fold you closely to my breast
To comfort you and give you rest...

If it were then, so long ago,
And you were young and did not know,

I'd tell you that you're brave and strong.
I'd hold your hand and sing a song

Of love and hope and things to come.
I'd buy a wagon and a drum!

I'd like to make the dreams come true
For that small boy who once was you...

1988

My Voice Swept Away on the Wind

I had a collie
when I was three.

Mother let me wander freely
through the fields —
knowing Collie would protect me
and bring me safely back.

One day Collie went out alone
and didn't come home again.
I remember standing in the doorway
    calling, calling, calling
        my voice swept away
                on the wind...

A neighbor told my dad
that he saw her near his sheep
and shot her.

Sometimes I think of Collie—
understanding clearly now
how things can be taken from you

and still I hear myself
    calling, calling, calling
        my voice swept away
                on the wind...

December 1992

In the Shadow of Hiroshima

Far away, I hear the drums
Beating, beating, beating...
They sound so sure.
An unknown fear clutches my soul.
Primitive terror turns my heart to ice
And jagged edges tear the tender flesh.

Nearer now, I hear the drums
Beating, beating, beating...
They sound so strong.
I see my fear grow in your eyes.
I see the smile fade from your lips.
Your face becomes still as in death.

Nearer yet, I hear the drums
Beating, beating, beating...
They sound so cruel.
You hold me close
As if there is no tomorrow.
We cannot know.
We dare not pray.

Never now, I hear the drums
Beating, beating, beating...
They sound no more for me.
I do not fear "the arrow that flieth by day
Nor the terror that flieth by night."
I shed no tears—nor laugh again.

There is no tomorrow.
There is no today.
There is no you...

1948

Kaleidoscope

My life is a kaleidoscope—

Will there always be
    too many pieces
        forever changing
            into lovely
        heartbreaking
    maddening
breathtaking
        patterns?

1967

Phone Call

I hear her jumbled words—
The shriek—
My heart turns to stone.
I know the fabric of our lives
Is forever changed.

I hold her in my arms
Through the long night
With passionate desire to
Protect her from the dawn
From the remembering that
He is gone.

Days, weeks, months
Drag slowly by....

It is not right,
It is not right,
I cry!

My daughter can't be
Widowed
Before I!

1975

Too Soon

I see you lying there
In a tangle of wires and tubes,
Long awaited child—
Cherished dream—

It's too soon, my love, it's too soon.

Your skin is dusky—
Your perfectly rounded little head
And tiny limbs turn blue.
I fight back tears.

The lights blink.
The monitor screams.
My heart stops.

Feverishly they work—
These masters of technology,
Holders of the healing arts,
Conveyors of compassion.

You can do it, little one.
You can live.
Silently I will you to fight.

We all want you—
Your mother who is so ill,
Your father who is so distraught,
Your brother who is only seven,
Your aunts, uncles and cousins,
Your grandparents and great-grandparents,
And friends you've never met.

It is such an assault to you—
The procedures,
The lights,
The noise.

I gaze at you,
Long awaited child—
Cherished dream—
Precious life—

Then I go back to your mother,
My long awaited child—
My cherished dream—

And silently will *her* to live.

1988

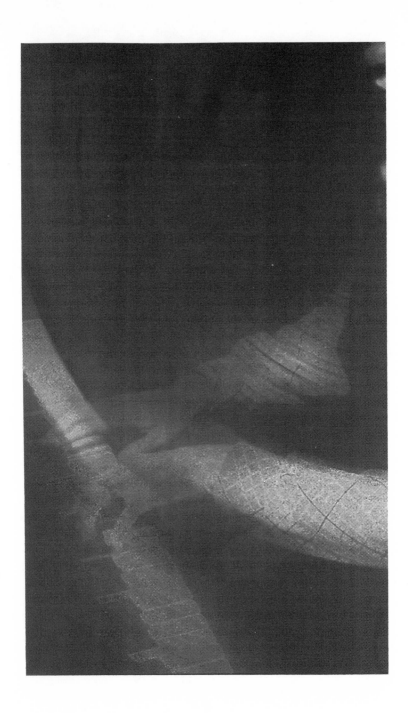

I Never Meant to Write a Book

You Cannot Break a Poet's Heart

A poet cannot be broken-hearted.

When a dear one dies, she writes a requiem
When a lover is untrue, she writes a sonnet
When the world is cruel, she writes satiric verse

A poet can take all the grief from her heart
(The pain that can swell and break a heart)
And write it in fine black lines
On starchy white paper

Oh, no, you cannot break a poet's heart.

1946

13

A Reflection on Fine, Black Lines

I wrote "You Cannot Break a Poet's Heart" the winter I was 16. I distinctly remember feeling quite pleased with myself, thinking that writing poetry endowed me with magical powers to triumph over fear and pain.

Now I see it was only a shadow of things to come—that it somehow reached into the core of my being to touch the woman who lived in that young girl.

And I see now, of course, I was wrong. Any heart can be broken. But I also see a grain of truth in the poem. The "fine black lines on starchy white paper" became a way to cope, to search, to travel toward understanding.

I wrote during the years I was a too-serious teenager, a very young bride, a not-quite-so-young mother and an even-less-young piano teacher.

I jotted thoughts on scraps of paper, napkins, and torn envelopes, and in my beloved diaries. But I never meant to write a book. Well, I *did* write one when I was 14. I copied the text very carefully with purple ink into a spiral notebook. But I didn't mean to write *this* book.

I simply wrote poems as lifelines of sanity. I wrote poems to celebrate, poems to clarify, poems to revisit sadness. Sometimes overwhelming emotion just spilled onto the paper as I reflected on events that I could not have written about when they occurred.

And I wrote poems in an effort to make sense of the Darkness.

I probably would have gone on indefinitely—writing a poem here, writing a poem there, tossing them into the battered box marked "Lois' Writing." But my life suddenly encountered several turns that were so startling and so unexpected that my search was intensified and my journey was altered forever.

CFS (Chronic Fatigue Syndrome) was the first jolt. On the morning of April 6, 1989, I had an unusual sense of well-being—renewal was evident in the cherry blossoms, the tender leaves, and the gentle warmth. I felt particularly well. But when I got up from a short nap at 3:30 p.m., I knew I was ill. I gave the evening piano lessons as usual. By the time I finished teaching, my fever was 104°. The desire to lie down was the strongest I had ever experienced, but I could not stand the weight of even a sheet on my body.

I assumed I had the flu. It didn't even occur to me to go to the doctor. I thought, I'll just stay in bed over the weekend and I'll be fine by Monday. After four days I felt a bit better and my fever had returned to almost normal, so I resumed my regular schedule—I didn't want to get behind, with the Spring Recital only six weeks away.

Six days later I awoke with more intense pain, weakness, and lack of motion in my hands, wrists, knees and ankles. I could barely pick up my coffee cup, walk to the bathroom or stay out of bed. By evening, a dense purple rash covered my legs from knees to ankles. The clinic nurse practitioner did not have a clue what was wrong. Neither did anyone else.

For five months I was periodically tested for Lyme disease and other possible causes for the continuing sore throat, headache, low-grade fevers, joint pain, overwhelming malaise and other assorted symptoms. In September my new internist diagnosed CFS.

I was relieved to have a name for the problem. I was not relieved to think of having something about which so little was known and for which there was so little help.

Aside from my husband and children, I told no one about the diagnosis for two years. I tried to hide my symptoms, rested on the sly, and made excuses so I wouldn't have to do so much. I felt a sense of shame in having an illness that was portrayed with such triviality in the media. CFS was dismissed as the trendy disease of the late 80's—the *yuppie flu.*

It felt neither trendy nor yuppie to me. I discovered what it is like to not know at 10:00 a.m. how I will feel at noon, to stand at the foot of the stairs and wonder how I will make it to the top, to be too tired to lift a pencil or hold a book, to have to rest two hours every afternoon and go to bed by 8:00 or 8:30, to play the piano and have a finger "lock up," to have to wear a jacket (even on a summer day) with pockets to carry my arms, and to forget an entire thought in the middle of a sentence.

When I was diagnosed with breast cancer a year later, I almost felt validated. At least everyone understood *that* disease and its implications. Almost everyone has heard of the terror, the incredible sense of loss, the fear of disfigurement and death.

There has been no way to sort out how much of my weakness and fatigue comes from CFS and how much has been caused by the cancer surgeries and treatments. I do know it is likely that CFS has caused at least some of the difficulty in recovery and some of the residual pain in the surgical areas.

And I know that writing has been a lifeline to reality and healing.

Still, I did not intend to write a book. But when I shared the writing with doctors, nurses and friends, they encouraged me to share my experience with a wider audience.

Sometimes I laugh and say I had three things to get off my chest—this book is the third!

July 1992
January 1993

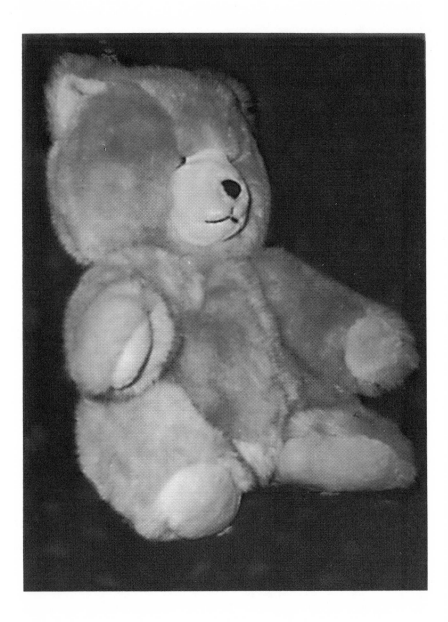

I Wish I Had
My Teddy Bear

January 1990

I feel caught in a web of aging and illness. I am so tired I can barely walk up and down the stairs. Sometimes I think I must be dying, but I know CFS is not life threatening.

February 11, 1990

Last night, snuggled under my blankets, I checked my breasts as I have done almost unthinkingly for the past thirty years [as automatically as I would lock the door and turn out the lights]. I was startled to touch two small "peas" that I knew had not been there before. I have checked so often that I can't imagine where they came from. [More than three years later, I still can't understand. And I am surprised I thought of the lumps as either *small* or *peas* —they were larger than dinner peas and as hard as pebbles.]

I have had cysts before—one even required a biopsy, but it was benign. I had a clean mammogram in November. So I dismissed the peas, rolled over and snuggled deeper.

March 8, 1990

My internist gave me an antibiotic for bronchitis, sympathized with my CFS symptoms and ordered a new mammogram when I casually mentioned the lumps. He promised to call before we go on vacation if anything shows up.

19

April 4, 1990

The mammogram was negative but the lumps are still there. The internist sent me to a surgeon. [I had been to see the surgeon in August because there was a clear fluid leaking from that nipple. He said then that many women experience galactorrhea and reassured me that I need not worry as long as the fluid remained clear. He also checked my breasts thoroughly—there were no lumps. The fluid has been discolored for a month or two now, but until today I hadn't made the connection.]

Thinking the surgeon might suggest waiting a few months to see if there would be a change, I marched in, planning to insist on a biopsy. But he did not reassure me this time. He told me that it was mandatory to remove the lumps as soon as possible. The tone of his voice sent a small shiver down my spine.

I asked to delay the surgery for two weeks since I'm committed to play the organ for Palm Sunday and Easter services at church. The news upset Les as much as it did me. We can't even think about it. Nor can we stop thinking about it.

April 20, 1990

Les and I went to the hospital and the two little peas were removed under general anesthetic. I had originally chosen a local anesthetic, but I think I didn't want to see the doctor's face.

After we came home from the hospital, I watched television awhile before I finally asked Les what the surgeon had said. Even before he spoke, I knew that I had cancer.

Les and the children are very upset, but I feel I must stay calm for their sakes. In our thinking and planning, we have always expected that I would live longer than Les. [He is eight years older.] Although I have given a lot of thought to widowhood, Les is struggling for the first time with the possibility that he could live longer than I.

April 21, 1990

I do not feel as calm tonight. Les and I just held each other and wept. I realized today that I will always be either a cancer victim or a cancer survivor. That ugly word is connected to *me*.

April 23, 1990

Les was gone today and I was alone with my thoughts. I am so scared. I am worried about the students. Karen [our daughter] called and she can't quit crying. Russ [our son who is a pathologist] predicts I will have to have a mastectomy. I cried and cried. I don't want to lose my breast and I certainly don't want to die. The outcome depends on what my body can do—the track record isn't too great so far.

April 24, 1990

The internist told me today not to take any more estrogen. Actually, I took my last dose the night before the biopsy, knowing that if I had cancer, I would have to quit. I think even then I knew deep down I had cancer.

April 25, 1990

I didn't sleep after 1:45 a.m. I am really suffering estrogen deficiency—insomnia, hot flashes, terrible night sweats, a very drawn feeling. It is disconcerting to face menopause for the second time at age 59. [I faced it with the same abruptness when I had a hysterectomy at age 36, but Estrogen Replacement Therapy interrupted the symptoms for the next 23 years.]

It is difficult to deal with logistics while suffering yet another body failure. I feel very upset about my teaching, because I have to be enthusiastic about the compositions the students are writing for the big recital next month and I don't even know if it will happen. I am not quite ready to tell them about the cancer, but meanwhile I feel I am living a lie. They will be so upset when they hear.

I hate having to change my life. I feel incredibly angry about this interruption. And I fear people will not relate to me in the same way once they know I have cancer. What *is* there about that word?

April 26, 1990

I started getting acne today. *That* didn't take long! I'm losing my complexion, my music, my disposition, my breast and who knows what else. The CFS is really kicking up—sore throat, achy joints and extreme fatigue. I'm trying to be brave and strong—to maintain the image I have of myself.

April 28, 1990

I cleaned the closets and drawers. I have such a passion to toss extraneous belongings. They all seem extraordinarily unimportant. Am I simply trying to control *something* in my life, even if it is the trivia? [In all the months since that day, I have been driven by a passion to keep my life clear of too many possessions, too many pieces of paper, too tight a schedule.]

May 1, 1990

Russ called today to report the information he had gathered from his colleagues at Duke University. It confirmed what I had already learned here. I made final arrangements for the surgery on May 7. Because there are two lumps, I need to have a mastectomy—but at least that way I can avoid the invasive treatment of radiation. My doctor said I had done an excellent job of research. I beamed like a schoolgirl. I feel like a schoolgirl—taking an exam in a course I did not choose.

Having put it off as long as I could, I went to tell my parents about the cancer. I hated to crush their belief that I will always be there to take care of them. My mother sat there frozen, too shocked to speak or cry. My father's stooped shoulders sagged even more.

May 3, 1990

It really sank in today that I will lose my breast. I'm grieving a lot over that loss and will continue to, I imagine. In spite of everything we had a pleasant, if poignant, dinner out. Later Les and I made love for the last time with my body intact. We wept and wept.

May 4, 1990

Les has reluctantly gone to a conference with Bob [our oldest son]. He didn't want to leave me alone, but I encouraged him to go. I told him I need solitude to deal with what is happening to me. I have to replenish my physical and emotional resources during the next two days so that I can face the surgery and help Les and the children deal with it, too. [I didn't stop to think that maybe he needed to be with me as much for his own sake as for mine.]

May 5, 1990

Keith [our middle son] called again today. I can hear the worry in his voice. Later, Karen came to be with me for several hours. We planned the music lessons she and Bob will teach for me next week, talked and hugged. It was something we both needed. I finally finished calling relatives, friends and each of my students—more than fifty calls in less than a week. Everyone seemed to appreciate the personal message.

I think I have it all together—I think I can bear to lose part of myself.

Goodbye, Beloved Breast

Goodbye, beloved breast
I shall never forget you—
Shall I ever come to the end of grieving?

When first you developed in sweet innocence
I was dismayed—
I was afraid of emerging sexuality...

But you became beautiful
My lover treasured you
My children nuzzled you and were nourished
I cradled you in my hands to cherish your softness...

Now a dark menace has invaded you
And somehow I must bear our parting...

Goodbye, beloved breast
Goodbye, beloved part of me
Goodbye, symbol of my femininity...

May 6, 1990

24

May 8, 1990

Being wheeled into surgery yesterday, knowing that what I had been resisting with every fiber of my being, was actually happening, turned out to be one of the more difficult challenges in my life. Other traumas had *happened* to us and we were left to deal with them. But I *made* this decision, and I was *letting* it happen, even though I felt like jumping off the cart to run screaming down the hall.

When I was first diagnosed with breast cancer, all I could think of was that I had known at least twelve women who had died of breast cancer, and I could think of only two who had survived. Since then, I have met *many* survivors and now know that when breast cancer is detected and treated early, the chances of five-year survival are 80% or better.

I had lost part of my body when I had a hysterectomy. I was surprised by how much I minded knowing that I would never again bear a child, but I did not experience the same loss then that I was anticipating now. For one thing, I had never cuddled my uterus, nor had I seen it. As much as I had tried to prepare myself, I had an absolute horror of losing that breast.

I awakened in the middle of the night, knowing that I shouldn't have sent the family home at 10:00 p.m. I just could not believe that I was lying in a hospital bed with my chest bandaged. I longed for my teddy bear.

May 9, 1990

This morning I finally could eat, and breakfast tasted good. But when I bathed afterward, I saw my chest for the first time and cried. They were gross—those fine, black surgical lines where my soft breast had been—and my poor remaining breast looked so alone. The 23 nodes that were removed showed no sign that the cancer had spread beyond the breast, but the pathologist did find an additional primary cancer.

25

I Wish I Had My Teddy Bear

I wish I had my teddy bear—
I could pretend that I am five

    clinging to my mother's dress
    knowing my father could do anything
    hearing fairy tales that ended
    "and they all lived…"

I wish I had my teddy bear—
I could pretend that I am thirty

    toddlers clinging to my dress
    believing their father could do anything
    reading fairy tales that ended
    "and they all lived…"

I wish I had the teddy bear
my husband gave me years ago—

    the day our last child left the nest
    even though neither of us quite understood
    why I wanted one

If I had my teddy bear—

    a little friend who listens well
    something to cling to in the night

Perhaps I would not feel so alone…

1992

26

It Is Rude to Interrupt
(When Someone Is Living)

An interruption to my life
    this body failure
    sense of doom

I cannot alter the tough facts
    just look at them
    just face them square

The barricade is simply there
    no way around
    one must push through

I hate this interruption
    the time it takes
    the time it steals

I feel anger, no control
    of my small world
    not at this time

The journey is so different now
    that I must find
    new paths to take

June 1992

June 4, 1990

We returned from a reunion with our children and grandchildren on the North Carolina beach. It was wonderful to be together, but I found it very painful to be in such a familiar setting and feel like such a different person.

Usually homecomings are very joyful for me, but not today. Did I somehow think that the magic of a vacation could magically erase the past two months?

The inability to lift even the baby, the jarring of the children's hard little heads as they tried to snuggle against my missing breast, the effort it took to walk with them looking for shells—all underlined my fragility.

I have such a deep sense of loss. I'm sure it is a time for growth, but I don't feel like growing.

June 11, 1990

I started radiation therapy today. The mastectomy was supposed to avoid radiation. But when the oncologist read the pathology report last week, he felt the third cancerous lump was too close to the surgical margin to take the chance. "If it had been five millimeters instead of only one…." So the breast is gone and electrons will invade my body, anyway.

June 24, 1990

This is the day we were to have left on a 38-day Super Grand Tour of Europe. [We had booked it in January, even though we were concerned about the CFS, thinking that we should try to go while we were still able.] I put on a pretty blouse, pinned a fluffy [falsie] on one side, and took a radiation treatment; then we ate at McDonald's.

I would have liked Europe better.

July 18, 1990

I had the last radiation treatment today. I am very glad to be finished. I will not miss the additional fatigue, the increased nausea, the burns.

Like a sunburn, the skin continued to redden, then blistered and peeled for weeks after the radiation stopped.

At the time, I didn't feel fortunate. But, looking back, I realize I was. The doctors hadn't had to interrupt the treatment because of the side effects. Some people suffer such severe burns during the course of their radiation therapy that they must stop awhile to let the tissue recover.

Chemotherapy sometimes destroys so many white cells that patients have to postpone their chemo treatments to give their bodies a chance to generate more cells.

They must be tortured with mixed feelings—glad not to be taking treatment, worried because they aren't currently doing something to fight the cancer, yet dreading the resumption.

But I will miss the kind people who have treated me. I wrote a farewell poem and left it with them today.

I also stood on my head before I left. I always stand on my head for each music class before summer vacation. The radiation therapists were amazed; the children take it for granted. One student told me twelve years ago [I was 47!] that she had never known such a little old lady to be so active. Or maybe she had never known such an active little lady to be so old....

Radiation

I lie on the hard table.
Calculations are made, angles are adjusted.
The tiny light above me blinks.
Lines of treatment
Are carefully drawn
On my chest.
Then the technologists are gone—
Gone with their friendly chatter,
Gone with the cheery "Here we go."

I am alone
In the round room
With the soft light—
Alone with the huge machine,
Surrounded by six-foot walls of concrete.
The machine hums
Then it begins to screech.
I slowly count the seconds,
Knowing there must be 45…

I wonder if the light is healing.
I wonder how my tissue will hold up.
Day after day
I enter the room with the machine.
Is radiation my friend?
Can it be my foe?

I count each day,
Knowing there must be 25…
One day I am finished.
The electrons have done what they can.
I go to resume my life.

It will be good again—
It will be filled with busy days.
Children will smile at me.

I will watch the sun rise and set.
But that tiny fear lurks
In a dark corner of my soul,
Ready to pounce
When I am tired
And the sun goes down...

July 1990

31

Last Day

Treatment is ended...

    a missing breast
    a fading scar
    a tangled network of nerve endings
    a residing pain and numbness
    a gnawing uncertainty

Life will go on, of course...

    but I will not
    be the same...

July 1990

Energy Crisis

At first I was energized

The diagnosis shocked me into action
The clutching fear galvanized me
The details demanded attention
The family's tears called for comfort
The decisions were made
The adrenaline flowed and I was energized

But one day all the energy was gone—
Physical, psychic, emotional—
The days turned into weeks
And the weeks into months

Now I search
Each cell of my body
Each corner of my mind
For
                one tiny spark

July 1990

July 23, 1990

Many years ago, while waiting in a doctor's office, I saw an article in *Reader's Digest* about making a commitment to keeping sex alive in marriage. It grabbed my interest, so I brought it home, and Les and I discussed it at length. We had always had a lively and passionate physical relationship, so it almost seemed ridiculous to make such a promise, but we did.

The promise has served us well over the years. We made our dates and faithfully kept them, working around Les's night shift for 26 years: when there were teenagers in the house, when time pressures overwhelmed us, when back surgery and a broken pelvis required some ingenuity.

The promise serves us well now—especially now. There are days when it seems almost hopeless to even try to keep sex alive in our marriage. The obstacles seem almost impossible to overcome—the lack of libido, the drenching hot flashes, the lingering surgical pain, and the feeling of ugliness that will not go away no matter how much Les reassures me that I am beautiful.

But by honoring our commitment, we still share tenderness, love, joy, and yes, ecstasy—especially ecstasy.

They'd Never Believe It

The young ones glance at us
and wonder
"Where's the glow?"

We smile and shake our heads—
There's no way
they can know!

1990

Good Morning, How Are You?

It's best to act normal—
To say "I'm just fine."
What everyone wants is
A positive sign.

Just smile and say thank you
When people will ask.
One mustn't let on that
Each day is a task.

Friends keep on calling—
You know they mean well.
But really they'd rather
For you not to tell

Each symptom, each detail,
Each wearisome day
Or mention that small fear
You can't drive away.

An illness gets tiring—
For them and for you.
The difference is simple—
They get to quit.

July 1990

Battleground

I am alive. The hell is done.
This early skirmish has been won.

And now it just remains to see
If further contest waits for me

If other shadows shall arise
And darkness once more cloud my skies.

The battles come, the battles go.
Live or die, I'll always know

My spirit can forever soar—
Already I have won the war.

August 1990

37

Small Amusements

There are some small amusements
Though at first they're hard to see
Like fluffing up my fiberfill
To make it look like me.

I have an empty pocket now
To store important things
Like passports and my credit cards
Or maybe diamond rings.

And there are times I have to smile
When people glance my way.
They stare and then get flustered—
They aren't sure what to say.

And once I had to chuckle as
A mirror I passed by.
My fluffy was off to the side
Its nipple much too high.

And exercise can bring a laugh
When I go out to trot.
One side is jogging with me—
The other side is not.

There are some small amusements,
But I find them very small.
And sometimes giggles turn to tears
And I can't laugh at all...

August 1990

38

Glimpse

I have looked at my mortality

Somehow that glimpse closes the gap
Between the here-and-now
And the once far-distant
Edge of tomorrow

It erases the perceived boundary
Between "if" and "when"

Time that once stretched endlessly
Has snapped
Like an old rubber band

I have always known that life is terminal—
But I did not understand it
Quite so well
Before

August 1990

The Gift

It is a gift—
    this reminder of mortality
    this thing that slows me down
    this reflective summer

I know things about myself
I could not otherwise have known—
    pain can be endured
    uncertainty can be tolerated
    loss can be processed

I know there is a well-spring of
    strength
    courage
    joy   within me

I know that time is not forever
There is
    an urgency
    a poignancy
    a preciousness   to life

I know that I do not fear
    suffering or death
    as much   any more

It is a menace
It is a sorrow
It is a loss of innocence
                 it is a gift

September 1990

40

To Les

You were the one who stood by me
You were the one who gave me
The news I did not want to hear

You were the one who held my hand
When they wheeled me into surgery
Yours was the first face I saw when I awoke
Yours were the tears that mingled with mine
When they removed the bandages

You were the one
Who never abandoned me
To lessen your pain

When I hurt and felt battered
It was your arms that held me
It was your hands that caressed me
It was your eyes that said
Even more loudly than your words
"You are still beautiful"

You were the one who stood by me
Through the terror, the pain, the healing—
Into love

You are the one I cherish
More than life itself—
My love and gratitude are
Beyond speaking

December 1990

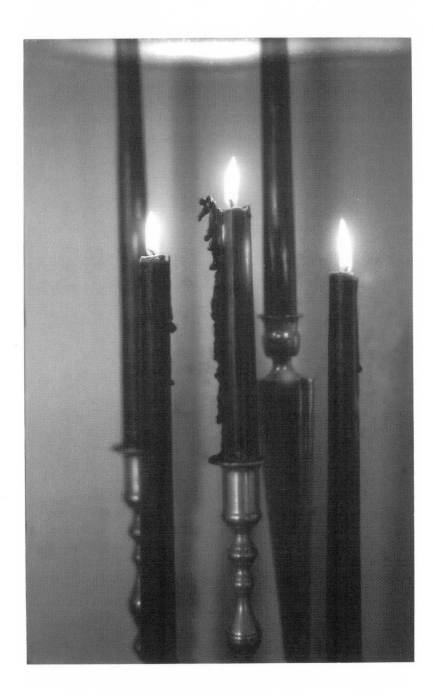

We Light the Lamps and Candles

First Call

I close my eyes this morning
While I soak in the tub—
Suddenly a tunnel of
Bright Light beckons me

I test the illusion—
    Close my eyes tighter
    Cover my face with my hands

Still I see
The Beautiful White Light—
I bask in warmth and peace

Then I turn back
And open my eyes

It is not time

November 1990

October 1990

We made our usual fall trip to see Keith and Russ [our sons who live out of state].

Russ took us to his pathology lab one afternoon and showed us my cancer cells through the teaching microscope. It was startling to see the enemy for the first time. I actually feel fortunate to have a missing breast.

Just Turn and Go

We went East again this fall—
The annual visit to
Our children.

As always it was good to see them
As always they were kind and gracious
As always we observed the rituals—
And pretended we did everything
As vigorously as before.

As always I learned more
About our children
Than I had known.

This time I learned
A new thing
About myself—

I can no longer
Bear to say
Goodbye.

October 1990

Map

I have developed

    a sense of place
    a sense of geographical location
    an awareness of where I am

        in time
        in space
        in history
        inside

perhaps it is
as important to know
where I am
as who I am

November 1990

Blurred Vision

I adjust the binoculars
And marvel at
The veins of the leaves
I can see in the distance.

I remember a recent time
When I could see clearly—
Colors were bright
Life stood out in precise relief.

Now everything seems
Slightly off-center—
The edges are fuzzy
The distance is blurred.

How could such a tiny
Shift in focus
Produce
This much vertigo?

October 1990
March 1993

November 3, 1990

It is six months since surgery. I had hoped I would be normal by now, but the fatigue and pain continue. When I feel fairly good, I plan excursions, events, projects. Sometimes I can pull them off—sometimes I can't. But there are other times I barely function.

Night after night I fall into bed exhausted. Occasionally Les even has to undress me. I wish it were as simple to remove the black fog that clouds my mind.

Paradoxically my teaching year is going exceptionally well. I think it is because I am concentrating on having fun with the students and on enjoying my work. The children distract me and give me mental and emotional respite, even as they wear me out physically.

I feel very torn trying to decide which people, events, and things are priorities. I am slowly realizing that I will not be going back to my old life.

When Daylight Has Gone

Sometimes when Daylight has gone
and tiny doubts play
in the shadows

I feel disheveled
my careful defenses unravel
a sense of sadness envelops me

Then I close the shutters to the world
I wrap myself in softest robe
I plump the pillows on my bed and

        quietly sink
     into the gentle comfort
       of the Night

November 1990

November 16, 1990

Today one friend told me that another friend had wondered aloud why I had not responded to her note, asking, "Doesn't she know the etiquette?"

I have received 187 cards and letters, plus beautiful flowers and gifts—a veritable shower of love. I wrote thank-you notes for the flowers and presents, but then simply had to make a choice between getting stronger and acknowledging each kindness.

I think of Ann, who is very ill, who feels she needs to respond to every card and letter. Sometimes she doesn't even open her mail because she knows she can't make the personal response she'd like.

It is painful for me to think of all the loving support she is missing in those unopened notes. It is painful, as I wonder what to do for her, to know that whatever I choose will only add to her burden. It is painful to see her use her strength by continuing to give to others, not realizing how much all of us would prefer that she rest or walk a bit in her garden.

Perhaps seeing Ann make such an effort to do more than even the most demanding etiquette dictates, at such expense to herself, has helped make my choices less difficult.

No Lifeguard on Duty

it is difficult
when one is drowning
to wave to the people
on shore

one wants to be
friendly, of course,

but perhaps it is
more important
to keep
swimming

.

December 1990

Eve's Apple

Let me treasure

    the not-knowingness of life
    the sense of uncertainty
    the wonder of worry

so I may hold close

    the preciousness of passage
    the awareness of being alive
    the freshness of the First Morning

1990

A Special Blessing

It is a special blessing
to have parents who have
grown old

I take comfort
in knowing the path ahead
can be trod with
    courage
        dignity
            grace

I find solace
in growing old enough myself
to observe and understand
parenthood from
three perspectives

I feel gratitude
that life has lasted long enough
(for them and for me)
    to bridge the gaps
        heal the pain
            return the love

It is a special blessing
to have parents who have
grown old

1991

December 14, 1990

My parents came to share a pre-Christmas supper with Les and me. I have been wondering what they are feeling about my illnesses—they who have stayed well for 84 years. They were visibly upset when I first told them about the cancer, but their Germanic stoicism served them well.

I asked them if they would write a page for me, describing their feelings. They were taken aback and Mother exclaimed, "Oh, my!" My father said he doesn't need to make a list—he can summarize it all with one word. When I prodded him, he replied, "Horrible." Mother added, "If you just think about *your* daughter having cancer, you will know how I feel."

I silently wondered if her answer were a way to avoid writing that unpleasant page—it is terrifying to realize you could outlive your own child. And I wondered if our feelings would really be the same. I am 60 and no matter how much I might wish to live many more years, I feel I have had a full life. On the other hand, *my* daughter is 39 and has two young children. I can *imagine* that having a daughter with cancer would be very unsettling for anyone, but I can't *know*. Try as one might, it is impossible to know how someone else might feel about anything. But I *can* hear the deep concern and love in her voice.

I may never get those lists, but I feel my facing cancer and their facing old age connects us with a thread of fear and a need for courage.

I wrote a poem and gave it to them (and to myself) for Christmas.

We Light the Lamps and Candles

(for Paul and Bertha Tschetter)

In the autumn of each year
As the days grow short and rare
We will light the lamps and candles
Of the memories we share

In the winter of the year
When the nights are very long
We can light the lamps and candles
And sing forth a haunting song .

In the autumn of our lives
As we wonder, so we yearn
To see many lamps and candles
Lighting each new step and turn

In the winter of our lives
When the days seem all too few
We still light the lamps and candles
And our spirits yet renew

In the darkest night of winter
Where is strength for going on?
We wrap our courage 'round us
We rejoice that Hope has found us
And we light the lamps and candles
As we wait the coming Dawn...

December 1990

55

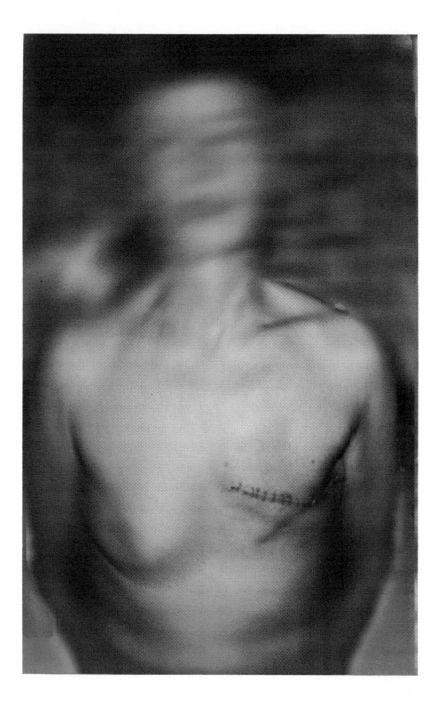

The author ten days after her first mastectomy.

I Have Looked
This Way Before

January 16, 1991

When I heard the news that the United States had begun bombing Iraq, I was crushed.

We had known since last August that events were propelling us in that direction, but I kept hoping against hope that somehow it would never happen.

My battle with cancer has changed my perceptions. Life has become so precious to me that I cannot understand how anyone anywhere could regard it as expendable.

January 20, 1991

I stayed home from church today, picked up my black pen, and spent the entire morning scratching my feelings onto paper. It was a way both to temper my pain and to share it with others.

War

History has shown
(since vision back is clearer
than vision fore)
that those who fight
and those who support
have often been deluded

And I
    who have fought battles of my own
    (sometimes valiantly, sometimes ungraciously)
    who have treasured the preciousness of life
    who have protested mortality fiercely

I feel an incredible sadness
    that humankind, alone among all species,
    with the power to reason
    with the ability to remember
    with the knowledge of consequences

is still sending its young
out to die

I can no longer endure
    man's inhumanity
    to man

January 20, 1991
March 12, 1993

Omniscience

As my knowledge increases
And I face my mortality—
I become more aware
I feel more pain

Yet...

No matter how hard won
I would not give up the knowledge
To lessen the pain
Always I long for a deeper awareness
Ever I yearn for fuller wisdom

Still...

I wonder...

Does the Enlightened One ever
Wish *He* didn't know?

And how does *She* bear the pain?

1991

Testing . . . 1, 2, 3

There it was—
A tiny drop of murky discharge
On my remaining nipple—

Will we now revisit
The vast wasteland of
Cancer treatment
As unwillingly and unready as the
First time?

Is this
Just a test
To see if we are still
Paying attention?

January 21, 1991

January 21, 1991

I am horrified by the Persian Gulf War. Now my consternation has been intensified by a personal horror.

The discovery that fluid is leaking from my remaining nipple [the first troublesome symptom in my lost breast] was a physical shock. I felt as if someone had kicked me in the stomach.

The first time I had the innocence of ignorance to protect me. There are *no* illusions now.

I want to focus on what I need to do next with as clear a mind as possible.

Knowing that I would see my gynecologist for a quarterly cancer checkup in four days, I reacted by immersing myself in work, tidying up my life.

I started with the photo albums which I normally update each January. But I didn't stop there. I got out the tiny cedar chest and sorted through letters up to fifty years old, reliving my life as I read them—the only letter I ever got from my father (explaining the solemnity of my upcoming baptism, the summer I was eight), incidental letters from my grandparents, the few letters that Les ever wrote to me (he hated to write), all the letters I had written to him during our courtship (I liked to write), letters from friends....

Then I cleaned out the memento drawers, creating a folder for each of my children. Next I tackled the income taxes and financial files.

Finally I opened the box where I had tossed all my poems for the past 46 years. I had meant to type and catalogue them some day. The time had come.

For ten weeks, while I was caught in the vortex of indecisive medical tests, an incredible feeling of urgency compelled me to press on, even when the energy and time my health allowed me were not enough. I had an insistent need to get my "paper project" put together! I wanted to make sense of those scattered pieces of my past.

In spite of my efforts to clear my mind by tidying up the pieces of my life, my anxiety continued. I wanted to ignore the situation. I couldn't see beyond a second mastectomy and what it might imply, so I wanted to stretch out my time as long as possible.

If I could stay awake until dawn—if I could just have one more summer...

January 24, 1991
My gynecologist did a test that was inconclusive and referred me to the surgeon whose regular appointment was coming up January 28.

January 28, 1991
The surgeon said there could be other causes for the discharge, but he ordered a new mammogram and checked me very carefully.

February 8, 1991
The surgeon called back today to say they couldn't see much by x-ray, but that that doesn't mean anything.

February 20, 1991
When I went for my monthly CFS checkup, the internist was pretty somber about the newest symptom.

February 26, 1991
"Mom," Russ called to say, "I have checked with my colleagues, and you only have two choices. You can watch, wait and worry. Or you can have the mastectomy now. A negative test will never *prove* you don't have cancer."

March 13, 1991
The nipple discharge continues. The oncologist found nothing in a breast check, but he said he couldn't say anything to allay my fears. He agreed with the others—as long as the symptom exists, I would *eventually* have to have a mastectomy.

April 19, 1991

The doctor was gentle and thorough as he put the needle into my nipple, threaded in the tiny tubing and took x-rays. As I lay there, I kept thinking, "Tomorrow is the anniversary of my first diagnosis of cancer."

The nurse kept her eyes on my breast. She said she couldn't bear to look at my face. The ductogram was excruciating—but it was not conclusive either. We will have to repeat the procedure next Friday.

The whole day seemed like "déja vu all over again." (Somehow it wasn't as funny as it was when Yogi Berra said it.)

One Year Ago Today

I am adjusted—
I am not reconciled

Fellow travelers
say I will be someday—

But I notice they never forget
the date of diagnosis—

April 20, 1991

Good News/Bad News

the good news is
there is no immediate
bad news

the bad news is
there is no way to guarantee
the good news

February 1991

You Will Be Just Fine

Please do not trivialize
My suffering.

You who are healthy
You whose mortality is as yet
Only dimly perceived—
Please do not say
"You will be just fine."

I may well be—someday—
But I do not know...
You do not know...

1991

Necessity

some things cannot be fixed
sometimes we simply
have to reinvent
our lives

February 1991

June 17, 1991

I have finally found a breast cancer support group to join. I felt I had come home as I walked into the roomful of women who *know*. But as I talked with them, I also felt the cloak of denial slipping to my feet.

The first few months after the diagnosis I was adamant that I did not wish to join a group. I was sure I wanted to "do it myself."

In the fall of 1990, about four months after my mastectomy, I sensed I wasn't handling things well and made some inquiries. But I wasn't willing to give up teaching for an entire afternoon and drive across the city during rush hour traffic to attend the one breast cancer support group I found.

My feelings of isolation continued to grow, however, and when I learned that a nearby hospital had a breast cancer support group, I found the courage to attend.

July 1, 1991

Since January the miserable ductograms, the other tests and the months of waiting have not detected cancer. But my second breast still leaks fluid [just as the first had]—no one feels confident there is no cancer. Mammograms did not pick up the previous cancers. By the time a new lump would be palpable, it might have spread to other areas of my body.

I have consulted with my own doctors and several others. Sometimes I feel as detached as if I were clinically discussing someone else.

I will have my second mastectomy July 8. This time I will take my teddy bear.

A Reflection on Gambling

It wasn't until I went to the support group that I realized I couldn't arbitrarily give myself a summer—I couldn't delay the second mastectomy until it suited me.

The group helped me realize that I was playing with my life. If I insisted on delaying the mastectomy until next summer, I was gambling with all my summers.

Since then I have seen other women also resist deciding—wanting a test or a doctor to decide for them.

In November 1992 a woman in our support group was struggling with a new threat of cancer. She had had many lumps over the years and a mastectomy in February. In October she had discovered three lumps in her other breast. And even though the triple biopsy was negative, she worried constantly that she would develop cancer in that breast, too. She didn't want to face her options—yet she continued to agonize.

One night in early November several women at the group finally asked her why she didn't consider a prophylactic mastectomy. She said, "I've just finished all my chemotherapy and radiation treatments. I just want to wait and see."

Although our situations were not really the same, I remembered my own struggle when I faced the prospect of cancer in my second breast less than a year after the first mastectomy. I pressed her: "You'd rather just wait until you have cancer again?" I felt terrible about having confronted her so directly. I could see she was upset.

But at the next meeting, she told the group, "I'm having surgery the day after Thanksgiving." She seemed as relieved as I was.

January 1993

Fortitude

I am grateful
my heritage includes
fortitude

It is helpful
when Life's events
require one foot
in front of
the other

July 1991

July 8, 1991

The surgeon held my hand until I went under. (Is anesthesia a bit like dying? You're pretty sure you'll wake up again. But you can't be certain. And you want someone to hold your hand.)

I drifted in and out all afternoon. I felt quite helpless because I could not move either arm nor lift myself, and there is just one little ridge of my back I can lie on. [I'm glad I didn't know that I would feel helpless for several weeks. Even after I could lift myself, I still slept on that one little ridge for months because of the discomfort.]

July 10, 1991

The internist reported no evidence of cancer in the eight random samples taken, even though there were some abnormalities. But it would have been easy to miss a microscopic seed. He added that he is still convinced that the mastectomy was inevitable and that by doing it now we had our best shot at eliminating the risk of metastasis. I feel undone tonight. It seems like a long way back.

July 14, 1991

I'm kind of losing it today. I just can't bear that I have no breasts.

July 16, 1991

Uncle George [age 78] called from Florida. "So they cut off both your tits—what will Les do now?" It seemed so insensitive, I couldn't even think of a reply. His laughter still rings in my ears.

The Gown

The cloak of denial
Has slipped from my shoulders—
The second breast will go.
The long-fought decision
Has been made.

I dress myself in courage
And go to the hospital.

The second breast is gone.
Once more I gaze downward
With tears in my eyes.
Once more the pain and the fear
Overwhelm me.

My courage lies
In threads
Upon the floor.

Soon I will gather
Each fragile fiber
        And weave it into
                A mantle of hope.

July 1991

Double Amputee

I have looked this way
Before—
Flat-chested, pencil-thin

When I was ten

Strange it is to seem
A sexless child
Again

(Too bad about
The graying hair
And slightly sagging chin)

July 1991

74

A Reflection on a Title

My friend Peggy suggested that I change the title of "Double Amputee" (then called "Second Surgery"). I was quite taken aback. I had never consciously thought of my surgeries as amputations. She had sensed, however, in reading the manuscript of the book and in our endless talks, that my feelings about the surgeries might be deeper than I was expressing.

Intrigued with her idea, I rushed to the dictionary to learn that *amputate* means to cut or lop off, but that *amputee* means one who has had a limb amputated. In discussing the definitions, we thought about the historical reasons such a distinction might exist. *Amputee* seems to reflect men's experiences. Until recently the only body parts that have been cut off have been limbs.

Undoubtedly, men have suffered more loss of limbs than women, if for no other reason than men have been involved more directly in war. And men have had more accidents because they have been allowed and expected to be more active. But the restriction of the term *amputee* to limbs belies not only the broader use of *amputate* but also the psychological truth of cutting off a breast.

I took the idea to the breast cancer support group for discussion one Monday evening. Most of the women were quite horrified that the issue would even arise. But several women ventured that they indeed felt their mastectomies were amputations.

We talked of how our culture has viewed breasts and how form has replaced function in much of Western Civilization. And even as we argued that losing a breast could not be compared to losing an arm or a leg, some interesting questions arose: How long did women have to fight for the right to choose a modified radical mastectomy over a complete radical mastectomy, let alone a lumpectomy over either of those? How many women walked around disfigured or with a falsie on the loose before an adequate prosthesis was invented, let alone breast reconstruction? How important is it to have our bountiful bosoms restored?

There are obviously different levels of amputation. Losing an arm or a leg generally has far greater consequence than losing a finger. But an amputated limb can be replaced with a prosthesis that allows some functioning. In fact, people have been fitted with artificial limbs that allow them to ski, bicycle, or even rock climb.

A breast can also be replaced with a prosthesis or reconstruction. However, neither of these simulates any natural functioning. If you are young when you lose a breast, you lose the ability to nurse a child. If you are past menopause, you lose the artifact of that experience. In either case, you lose the pleasure of cradling a child to your bosom and the pleasure a breast brings to you and your mate during sex.

A prosthesis or reconstruction is only superficial. It looks good—score one for beauty pageants—and fills a void in your clothes.

But reconstruction *is* fascinating. You can have darling little nipples put on, complete with tattooed areolas around them. Sometimes after our breast cancer support group meeting, we go into the rest room to check out the newest scars and cute nipples. Sometimes we giggle like girls. Sometimes we cry.

But if a mastectomy is not an amputation, why was I so distressed at even the *thought* of losing my breast? Does choosing to have reconstruction help deny the concept of amputation and the constant reminder of cancer?

Several women and one woman's husband have told me that it was very important to them to begin immediate reconstruction, returning from the operating room with little mounds already in place.

What makes us want to keep all our parts, sometimes even at the risk of dying? Years ago, I had a friend who had cancer in her leg. She said, "I would rather die than have my leg removed." And she did die, in fairly short order. In *Lonesome Dove*, a wounded cowboy said the same thing and paid the same price.

I have not heard of any woman who would rather die than lose her breast, but I would not be surprised if there are such women.

I certainly know that if I had to choose between losing a breast and losing an arm or a leg, I would sacrifice the breast.

But that awareness does not belie the fact that, deep inside, a part of me feels I am an amputee.

January 1993

The Mall

I went shopping today
    for a bra that would not bind
    for prostheses to remind.

It is difficult to search for something
    that you never really wanted
    in the first place.

July 1991

Force of Habit

Once before we went to sleep
my husband reached
to caress my missing breast—
I felt him cringe
and he slowly
withdrew his hand,
hoping I had not noticed.

Having done so once,
he never forgot again.

I learn more slowly.

Whenever I run up the stairs
my hands instinctively
fly toward my chest—
forgetting, after all this time,
there is no need to steady breasts
that lie on the cutting room floor.

March 1993

A Reflection on Losing My Breasts

When I had the first surgery and wrote "Goodbye, Beloved Breast" [p. 24], I was proud that I was facing the issues of grieving. I know now that I protected myself to a degree. I didn't realize then how much my bosom *was* a connection to the remembrances of my life as a mother, a wife, a nurturer.

Losing the breast was almost like losing a photograph album of our children when they were young. The breast was a connection to their infancy and childhood. It was the source of their earliest nourishment; the pillow upon which I rocked them to sleep; the cozy haven they burrowed into when they were hurt or scared.

My bosom was also a haven for Les—a place to rest his head when a day had been too long or a night became too sleepless. And then, of course, it was a symbol of shared intimacy—no, it was more than a symbol—it was a source.

Had I allowed myself, I might have wondered if the relationships would be diminished by this loss, if the memories would be tainted. I know now that I lost much more than a piece of cancer-invaded tissue. I compensate—but some things are irreplaceable.

The loss was most intense when I had the first surgery. The remaining breast was not much of a pillow or a haven. As for being a sex symbol, when we looked at it, all Les and I saw was *cancer*—a symbol of everything that threatened our happiness.

July 1991

80

Affirmation

The breasts are gone
But I am
Whole

Disfigurement
Need not include
My soul

August 1991

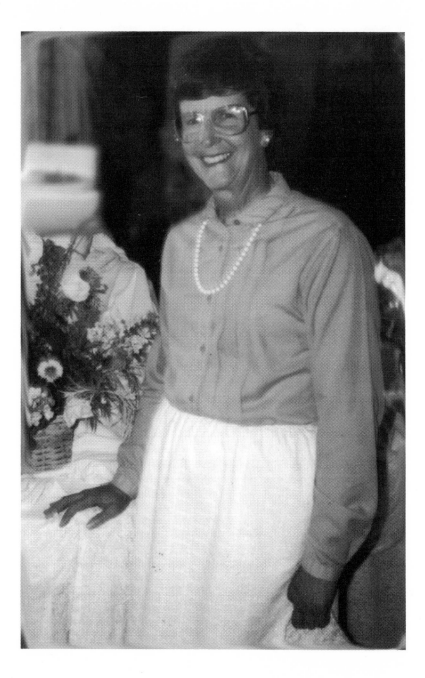

Ann Keener (September 22, 1934–August 28, 1991)

Hard It Is to
Lose a Friend

August 2, 1991

My dear friend Ann is losing her long battle.

She was diagnosed with breast cancer in May 1987. Her prognosis was grim from the beginning, but she fought valiantly and life went on. In some ways it seemed her life was good again, but she never really said so, and she never quite seemed her old self to me. Both of her once-slender arms had been distorted by lymphedema—swollen twice their normal size. And her eyes looked sad.

Then stomach cancer was diagnosed in March 1990. I felt devastated for her, and I gave her the poem "What Can I Say?" the day before her stomach was removed. When I was diagnosed with breast cancer in April 1990, Ann thought of me, not herself.

She called me today to come say goodbye. Remembering how much my teddy bear had comforted me the night after my second mastectomy three weeks ago, I took Courageous Lion to her. She immediately drew him close.

I assured her that I supported her decision to refuse the intravenous feedings, even though we both knew what that meant. I could see she felt peaceful and that has continued to sustain me.

Even so, my heart was breaking as I said goodbye and helped her plan her funeral. She told me her favorite composers, pieces of music, choral selections, scriptures, and whom she wanted to participate. I promised I would take care of it—somehow I will find the strength.

After Ann died, her husband was exhausted and distracted. When I offered to handle all the details for the service, he conceded: "What I need for this job is a good anal-retentive German!" (We both chuckled at his description of me.) It was more than I had promised Ann, and I don't know where I found the energy. But arranging her service was the only thing I could do for her, and it was the last thing I would ever do for her.

My oncologist later said he thought it was a courageous thing for me to have done, but I think not. I believe her asking me was a gift. It helped me deal with The Final Dark that awaits us all.

What Can I Say?

(for Ann)

What can I say to you, my friend?

You who are
    beauty
    compassion
    gentleness

You who have
    soothed
    comforted
    taught
    inspired

We have gone through much together
We have talked and laughed and cried
The days, months, years
Become a blur of sharing and of love

What can I say to you, my friend?
As you face again the
    pain
    fear
    uncertainty
    of cancer

Shall I say
    Keep up your courage
    (you who have been so courageous)?
    Keep up your strength
    (you who have been so strong)?

But we know that courage sometimes falters
And strength is not always ours to grasp

What can I say to you, my friend?

Perhaps I shall say nothing—
    I'll press you to my wounded breast
    hold you ever in my thoughts
    and hope you know how much I love you...

March 1990

Questions

(for Ann)

How do you live
when your life has been
reduced to dying?

Where do you find
some shreds of joy
amidst the crying?

When is it time
to cut the bonds and
give up trying?

1991

Shoreline

(for Ann)

Everything seems
so distant
now.

Is Life receding
or
is Eternity approaching?

1992

The White Horse

(for Ann)

Death comes on a white horse
to carry you away

I see the love in Her eyes as
She lifts you carefully
and cradles you in Her arms

You go willingly, eagerly,
even though you know

You can't come home again

August 1991

With Right of Survivorship

(for Ann)

Hard it is to lose a friend
Whose dying could foretell my end

And hard it is to pick up strands
Of living, when those other hands

Are stilled which often soothed my brow
And gave me courage up to now.

There is no way to understand
Why she is gone—and I am here.

September 1991

Farewell

(for Ann)

we will embrace
again some day

part of my soul
goes with you

and part of yours
will stay

September 1991

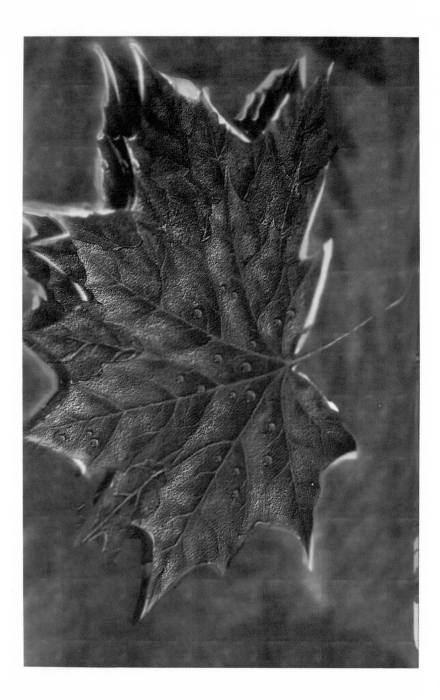

The Leaves Are Crisp Beneath My Feet

Autumn

I love to walk in autumn
Through deep woods
And bracing air—
The leaves are crisp
And crunch beneath my feet.

My heart is brittle, too,
As though it may disintegrate with
Any more beauty or
Remembered pain.

1978

September 1991

The women in the breast cancer support group struggle with how much to share about their cancer with people at work. Some have taken several months' leave of absence for treatment, carefully guarding their secret. [People tend to react in one of two ways—distancing themselves, as if cancer were contagious, or being oversolicitous, as if a cancer victim is totally incompetent.]

I began this teaching year unable to wear a prosthesis of any kind since I am too sensitive to wear a bra. I was worried about my obvious flatness.

The boys in the studio are probably too young to think much about it, and the adults can handle it. But I was concerned about how the girls would respond. I felt they would really wonder. [A year later, in a conversation with my twelve-year-old granddaughter, I knew my worry had been justified. She asked many perceptive questions and one of them was, "Are these little lumps growing on my chest *cancers?*"] I worried that the girls would think more about the cancer if I didn't wear a camouflage—I wanted somehow to protect them from feeling an ugly threat to their own budding breasts.

I decided to continue the openness I have always shared with my students. I answered their questions and explained that my chest is still tender, so I will have to be flat for awhile if they don't mind. Since they are already used to my many idiosyncrasies (one being the continual putting on and taking off of sweaters due to the hot flashes), they nod their heads knowingly and matter-of-factly say, "Fine, Mrs. Hjelmstad."

So much for worrying about *my* workplace.

End of Season

There comes a moment
when it is time
for summer to be over

There comes a day
when we must face
the winter
of our lives

September 1991

October 30, 1991

As a child, I often thought about dying—wondering how it would be, wondering where I would go—never quite able to imagine a world that didn't include me.

Thoughts of death continued to trouble me as an adult. Try as I would, I was never able to picture the world without me in it somewhere.

The diagnosis of cancer changed that. And for a long while, my glimpse of the world without me was extremely unsettling.

As we traveled across the country this fall, I pondered the lifelong questions again. As the miles and the days sped by, I became aware of another shift in focus. Somehow, without realizing it, I have begun to be at peace with my mortality.

Without Me

I'm not as attached to living
as once I was

Make no mistake—
I prefer to be alive

But

Sometimes now
I can imagine life going on—
without me

October 1991

Afterlife

Someday there will be
A tunnel of Light

I will find it and
Walk toward it

At the very least
I may find   cessation

I hope
I may find   joy

I am willing
to find   what is

1991

I Have Faith

If this life
is all there is
I have faith
that I have done
enough good
and little enough harm
to justify
my existence

And if another life awaits me
I have faith
that I will participate
as eagerly as I have
in this one

1991

Benediction

autumn lays
her gentle hand—
    a benediction
    o'er the land

October 1991

A Reflection on Positive Thinking

My friend Jack has faced many hardships over the course of his life. He has learned to cope by deciding that reality is only what you perceive it to be. The problem is that he has difficulty accepting the fact that other people do not always perceive reality the same way he does.

His commitment to positive thinking is certainly sincere, but sometimes he sabotages the effort of others to work through their pain in their own ways. Rather than trying to help people deal with their honest emotions, he sometimes refuses even to acknowledge them.

People often charge cancer (and other) patients to "think positively." Meaning well, some even give us books that become oppressive with hints that we are responsible for becoming ill and for getting well again.

"Push away that negative thought!"
"Oh, please don't say that!"
"If you think something bad, it will happen."
"With that attitude, it's no wonder you have cancer."
"If you really wanted health, you'd be well."
"You must think positively."

I have had several friends who heard and read similar things and who worked very hard to maintain an optimistic attitude in the face of some very discouraging facts. Eventually they all died—each having to deal with more than a destroyed body. I admired their courage, but felt very sad that they bore this additional burden.

Sometimes when I tried to break through the barrier, to get them to talk about what they were really thinking and feeling, they seemed afraid to even mention the possibility of not getting well, as though that would be a jinx.

Did they think they were causing their illness? Did they blame themselves for not thinking positively *enough*?

101

I believe there *is* a mind-body connection. Our attitudes certainly affect the quality of our lives. I very much believe in living in a positive way. My game plan has been to carry on my life, continue as much of my teaching and writing as possible, enjoy every moment I can.

But I also believe in reality. And regardless of what the best approach might be for others, I have found that facing limitations, accepting them, and working around them has helped *me* to cope.

It works out better some days than others.

November 2, 1992

Bed of Nails

if you lay
a blanket of joy
over everything

the spikes keep poking through

perhaps it would be better to
flatten the points
first

1991

November 16, 1991

The breast cancer support group has talked a great deal about "chemo" [chemotherapy]. As they catalogue the side effects—hair loss, blurred and changing vision, mouth sores, headaches, dry eyes, loss of concentration and memory, vertigo, sore glands, joint pain, loss of appetite, nausea, deep fatigue—those of us who have not had chemo sit on the sidelines. We don't know whether to feel lucky or undertreated. We sometimes feel embarrassed that we haven't been sick enough.

I went to the support group meeting for Chronic Fatigue Syndrome patients at National Jewish Hospital this afternoon. We heard an interesting lecture by a doctor from University Hospital. One thing particularly caught my attention—certain chemotherapy drugs produce many of the same symptoms as CFS. I haven't had chemo, but I do have CFS.

As I listened, I realized that my empathetic feeling for the chemo patients is medically sound—I *do* understand some of what they are experiencing!

After the meeting I asked the lecturer about the continuing pain and raw nerve endings I have in the surgical area. He said that it is quite common for CFS patients to experience ongoing pain after any kind of surgery.

Somehow it helps to know a reason, even though it doesn't lessen the pain.

On Dealing with Limitation

My life has been circumscribed
By the aspects of
    pain
    fatigue
    treatment

My priorities are
A series of nested circles
Beginning with the center
That is me

Daily I choose
The farthest orbit
I can reach
Daily I carefully
Spin out rings—
    nutrition, rest, exercise
    work, play, relationships

But what I really want is
To go zooming out
To the edges of my life
And dance on the periphery

1991

The Phone Lines Are Down

It is difficult enough
to process my emotions

to say nothing of
expressing them

November 1991

Badge of Courage

(to Les)

When you are gone
(if you go first)
there will be no one
    who has witnessed the struggle
    who will validate my badge of courage
    who can notarize the signature of pain

Where will I find
confirmation
of my suffering?

November 1991

Maturity

I have longed for Certainty.
I have cried for Truth.
I have sought the unimpeachable Faith.

I have wondered—
How would I know
If and when I found
The Answer,
Whether I had indeed asked
The Question?

Perhaps maturity is
Knowing there are no answers

And finding the courage
To live without them.

1991

Future Shock

In Nineteen Hundred Ninety-One
When I was feeling ill,
I put my papers all in shape
And codicilled my will.

I audited my earthly life;
I sorted and I tossed;
I mucked through papers endlessly.

I found my life and lost
My chronic fear of growing old
Or dying much too soon.

A rare and curious peace lay o'er
My empty, tranquil room.

And now it's Twenty Twenty-Eight.
The cosmic joke is mine!
Somehow the laughter's loud and long—
I'm almost ninety-nine!

March 1991

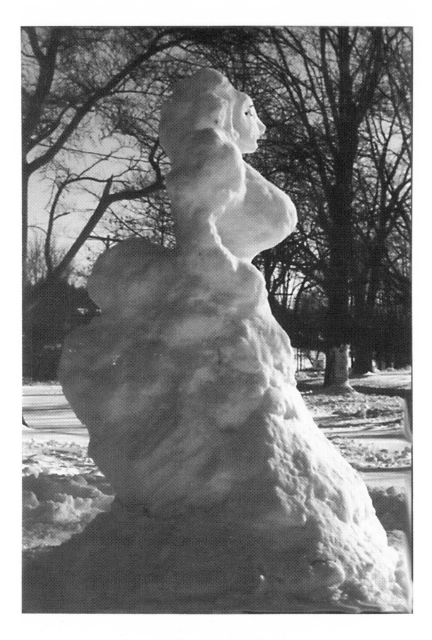

"Snow Lady" – sculpted and photographed
by Jim and Peggy Cole

I Cannot Help but Wonder

A Matter of Perspective

It was not until I had lost a breast myself that I began to notice how incredibly breast-oriented our culture is.

I couldn't open a newspaper without pages of lingerie ads staring back at me. I couldn't leaf through a magazine without seeing pictures of women who were scantily clad. I couldn't watch a television program without gasping for fear a bosom would fall out over the top of a dress.

Some days I look at women's breasts and think very detachedly, "Those are funny looking things. They are so foreign to me." If I had not taken pre-mastectomy photographs as part of my grand scheme to say goodbye properly and be done with it, I would not even remember what my bosom once looked like. Most mastectomy patients don't think to take such pictures. Some later wish they had, even though they know how painful it would be to see them.

On other days I think, "I would die to have them back." Then I laugh uncomfortably at the irony, realizing that I would indeed die if I had them back—particularly the one.

February 26, 1992

The results of my bone density test are in. The lack of Estrogen Replacement Therapy (ERT) has affected my bones as well as my skin, my vascular system (hot flashes and chills), my sex life, my ability to sleep, my sense of well-being. Will I get a dowager's hump and bowlegs? Will I break a hip?

It isn't just the new diagnosis that unnerves me. It is the domino effect. Did 23 years of ERT increase my risk for breast cancer? The issue is still controversial. But there is no question that the withdrawal of ERT contributes to osteoporosis. And post-menopausal women who are without estrogen rapidly develop the same risk men have of dying from a heart attack.

The recommended prevention and treatment for osteoporosis is eating foods high in calcium, taking calcium supplements and doing weight-bearing exercise. But I've been doing those things religiously for years!

Now, for two weeks out of every third month, I will take a medication that sometimes prevents additional loss of bone. We probably don't know the long-term side effects of that drug either.

Sometimes I feel like getting on my hands and knees and pleading for estrogen. But I don't believe I could bear thinking that it might feed an undetected cancer in my body.

I know that everyone eventually dies of something, but I will continue to fight each new threat to my health with as much knowledge as I can find and as much perseverance as I can muster.

On the other hand, I cannot help but wonder where it will all end.

Bone Loss

The tests show
I have osteoporosis.
The doctor seems surprised.
I am dismayed.
I feel betrayed again—
Alienated from my body—

I was counting on
My bones to hold me up
The rest of my life.

February 1992

113

Checkup

The checkups still cause
a tightness in my chest—
a primal fear

Every three months
the doctors poke and question—
 Any bone pain?
 Appetite OK?
 Muscle weakness?
 Headache?
 Nausea or vomiting?

Every six months
the lab tests and x-rays question, too—
 CBC?
 CEA?
 LDH?
 CA 15-3?
 Shadow on the screen?

Each time I pray for
"within normal range"

and wonder
what I will do
if the answers
are wrong
again

June 1992

Recurrence

I could live
the rest of my life
without it.

But if cancer recurs
can I count on
the recurrence of
hope and courage too?

1992

May 18, 1992

I need to make the final decision today whether to mail the student registration forms for the coming year.

The big Spring Recital was yesterday at the church with all 41 [of my piano] students participating, playing their own compositions and joining one another in ensembles.

Karen and Carl, Bob and Vicki, Keith and Kara, and Russ and Sandy [my children and their spouses] gave me a lovely reception afterwards in commemoration of my thirtieth anniversary as a music teacher.

It was a beautiful, festive afternoon. I felt most honored.

When I was diagnosed with cancer in May 1990, I feared that we would have to cancel the Spring Recital that year and I wondered whether I would be able to open the studio in the fall. When I had the second mastectomy in July 1991, the question arose again.

I wanted desperately to complete thirty years and that goal kept me going. But now that I have completed the thirty years, I have been wondering whether I should continue. CFS and the biopsies and mastectomies have sapped my strength.

Working with children depletes my energy—but it also very much revitalizes me. I am not sure how I will know when it is costing too much. It is a fine line.

For now, the balance still tilts in favor of the students.

Judgment Call

I am willing to spend a day teaching children
But I am not willing to track investments.
It was one thing when I had
All the time in the world.
It is another thing now.

I am willing to cook a tasty meal
But I will not wait to be served in a restaurant.
It was one thing when I had
All the patience in the world.
It is another thing now.

I am willing to listen to another's pain
But I am not willing to chit-chat over lunch.
It was one thing when
Any subject interested me.
It is another thing now.

I am willing to walk two miles in the woods
But I am not willing to hunt for a bargain.
It was one thing when I had
All the strength in the world.
It is another thing now.

I am grateful to discover the difference
Between things that matter to me—
And things that do not.

1992

Adventure

I have not known
much big adventure

I have lived in the same house
for thirty-three years

We have raised four children
    redecorated a bit
    driven about the country
    and made one trip to Europe

But basically—

I have spent the past thirty years
    surrounded by the same four walls,
    two blackboards, table, chairs,
    four pianos, stacks of music,
    generations of children

And yet—

Could I more adventure find
    than working with the heart and mind
    of young and gentle humankind?

1992

Pipe Organ

I am not a large woman
        and I am aging

I have been diminished by
        cancer
        surgeries
        chronic illness

But when I sit at the console
And my fingers touch the keys

        My spirit soars

Here—in the glorious sound—
        My muted voice
            sings again
        My faded beauty
            sparkles once more
        My waning strength
            shakes the rafters

1992

A Reflection on Friday Mornings

I have always loved laundry days, even on vacation: the hum of the washer and dryer, the fragrance of freshly washed clothes, the joy of patting the neatly folded stacks—the feeling of being connected to women across the centuries.

And I have always loved trying on clothing, assembling new outfits, coordinating color and texture, smiling at the reflection in the mirror, like a little girl playing "dress-up."

I often spend the time between loads of laundry experimenting with my wardrobe. And since my first mastectomy I also experiment with little bags filled with rice, rolled up pantyhose, rounds of polyester fluff, "Reach to Recovery" prostheses, permanent prostheses—all in an attempt to restore my body image.

Friday after Friday I struggle to get it right. The swelling, tenderness, and permanent nerve damage under my arms make me reserve the mastectomy bra with the beautiful $600 silicone mounds for special occasions like the wedding of a son.

Something within me rebels at hanging an uncomfortable harness on my frame—just so I can put something uncomfortable into it, so that I can feel that those around me are not uncomfortable being reminded of my mortality.

I went braless, breastless and fluffless for about two months while the initial healing took place. I'd look in the mirror and think, "I don't look so bad—no one can even tell." But one day a photograph made me realize that the flat chest wasn't as unnoticeable as I had hoped. I resumed my quest for a solution.

Currently I wear my own invention—little pockets which I sewed on the inside of an undershirt and fill with $4 falsies. It was more difficult when I had one natural breast to try to match, but sometimes now I forget exactly where the imposters should be placed.

The image in the *mirror* passes inspection. But the image of wholeness in my *mind* dissolves again and again. Will the image in my mind ever match the image in the mirror?

March 1992

The Walk

I struggled through
my walk today
each step a test
of determination

I was halfway through
before I even noticed
there were no clouds
in the sky

(I remember when
my morning walk
was the highlight
of the day)

April 1992

Journey

When the scenery is breathtaking
the weather a whisper of gentle warmth
the road clear

One almost wishes to
never arrive

When it is cold and rainy
when tiredness aches into the bones
and the horizon is obscured

The end cannot come
soon enough

June 1992

July 2, 1992

Our dear friend Ivan died today, less than six weeks after his diagnosis of pancreatic cancer. He is the first person in our close-knit church support group to die. We have been together 23 years. We all are devastated.

When he first heard the grim news that he had terminal cancer, he commented sadly, "I had always planned to be a very old man." He said he had never imagined that anything bad could happen to him.

Ivan's death, coming so soon after Ann's death, makes me wonder if death is ever fair. I am struck by the contrast between their deaths. I think that death came almost too late for Ann—allowing her body to be tortured. But for Ivan, it came too soon—hardly serving any notice at all.

Death Came Too Soon

(for Ivan)

Death came too soon.
The White Horse galloped
to the gate
and demanded
that you go.

"I am not finished!" you cried.
"I plan to be a very old man!"
But Death insisted
until you whispered
"I will go."

And we—
We are
      stunned by the swiftness
      numbed by the knowledge
      halted by the heaviness

We miss
      your historical perspective
      your political passions
      the twinkle in your eye
      your infectious chuckle
      your loving touch

Death came too soon, dear friend.

Yet at the end—
We felt your spirit soar away
And could not call for you to stay!

July 1992

August 3, 1992

Anger erupted at my cancer support group tonight. When it finished, the pile in the center of the room was impressive. There were many faces to the anger.

Ellen was angry that she had to change a perfectly good life to accommodate fatigue and treatment.

Harriet was most angry about losing her hair—when she took off her wig to show us, she looked like a survivor of Auschwitz. She calls her bald head a relentless reminder.

Beth was furious that her sisters refuse to talk about her illness—wanting her to put it all behind her, seeming to deny both the chronic aspect of the illness as well as the increased threat to themselves.

Cindy's marriage is crumbling. Among other things, her husband expects her to wait on him as she always has, even though her priorities have changed.

Liz continues to feel betrayed by her body.

My own anger had spilled out about a year ago as I watched Pavarotti in the Park on PBS [shortly after my second mastectomy]. When he sang the beginning note of "O Sole Mio" in that incredibly clear, controlled voice, my defenses suddenly shattered. Tonight as I listened to these women, I looked back on all the things I had been angry about.

My body has betrayed me, too. I had always felt that no matter what happened—loss of job, financial disaster, bereavement—somehow I could make it. I often said, "If you have health, you have everything." I have followed a healthy diet. I have walked three to five miles a day. There is no history of cancer in my family. Was it the Estrogen Replacement Therapy? Did I mismanage stress in my life? Even asking myself these questions makes me angry—they imply I caused my own cancer.

I was also angry with the answers to my medical questions: "There are too few studies on that issue to give you definitive information....We don't know what the long-term side effects of tamoxifen will be....We're not sure yet how your bones and heart could be affected...." I understand much better now that medicine is an art, not a science. I have received excellent and loving care—but *why* doesn't someone find out why one out of every eight women gets breast cancer?

I was angry that my family was trying to *make* me be well so they could return to their fantasies of life as it used to be: my husband wanting me to go out to dinner; my parents and my siblings wanting me to be the one they could all depend on; my daughter longing to have leisurely talks together again; my sons assuming the entire episode was over.

I was upset when they didn't understand my limitations. I have since realized I am not angry with my family—I am angry that my illness has caused so much disruption to their sense of well-being. I am angry with myself—I feel I have let them down.

I am angry that I have had to make so many choices between "not enough" and "way too little." Why should it have to be a choice whether I go out for lunch or follow my afternoon teaching schedule; whether I help my grandchildren build a sand castle or stay up for supper; whether I serve soup (when I wanted to make Chicken in Orange-Almond Sauce) to my guests or not invite them at all?

I can see that all of us (the members of my cancer support group and our families) are angry at having to change—at having to face our mortality and the loss of loved ones. Our routines have changed; our body images have changed; our relationships have changed; our perceptions of life itself have been profoundly altered.

But in spite of the pile in the center of the room, anger is *not* uppermost at many of our meetings. I have written many poems that are *not* angry. And I have reflected many times on why this is so.

Is it because most women "do guilt" better than we "do anger"? Is it because I spent so many years learning to cope with anger, that I no longer repress it until it erupts? Is it because I know all people have problems that I ask, "Why not me?" instead of "Why me?" (It amazes me to hear other people ask "Why me?" as if they feel they are somehow exempt from misfortune.)

Is it because the process of writing poetry, while it clearly does not prevent broken hearts, does release my frustrations?

Or have I simply learned that railing against the inequities of life requires more energy than I am willing to spend on a pile of shit?

Support Group

courage ebbs, flows

anger flashes, dissipates

love holds us together

August 1992

A Reflection on Commitment

Breast cancer is hard on the men in our lives. They must deal not only with the fear of losing us, but also with the tedium and trauma of treatments and our shifting moods as we confront our mortality. *We* often pull away from *them* because we cannot bear the possibility of rejection.

They must also deal with anger—ours as well as their own. They may be angry at feeling afraid we will die, angry at having their lives disrupted, but, perhaps most of all, angry at standards which say a man should not share his feelings with anyone—let alone a wife who is ill.

The men respond to the challenge in various ways—some not so noble.

Some men could not be more caring—accompanying us to treatments and consultations, seeing past our shrillness to the underlying fears, and cooking dinner when life is more than we can bear. Les told me that the husband of another cancer patient recently asked him, "How do you cope when your wife becomes irritable?" Les responded, "It's difficult sometimes, but I try to understand the reasons for it."

Some men become impatient and want to get back to life as usual: "You've had your surgery. You've finished your treatment. Now let's get back to normal!"

Sometimes conflicts arise from different ways of coping. One husband shared with Les his despair that when he expressed a desire to make love, his wife retorted, "I'm thinking about *death*—and you're thinking about *sex*?" She didn't understand his need for intimacy, and he didn't understand her fear of mortality.

Some men were never attached emotionally at all. Others withdraw emotionally when they can no longer bear to watch our suffering or when the fear of loss becomes unmanageable.

And some men respond the way the husband of one of my friends did. One day, he simply announced, "You have totally worn me out with your surgeries and treatments." Then he packed his bags and left.

Some of the women in my cancer support group have said they cannot imagine coping with cancer without a supportive man in their lives. Others have said they are grateful they only have to worry about themselves. I am sure that sometimes it would be easier to cope without having to consider the feelings and needs of a mate, but I feel fortunate that Les has been so supportive.

There is no question that breast cancer is a crisis in most relationships. It magnifies the strengths and weaknesses that already exist.

Les and I have always invested a lot of effort in our marriage. We realize we have to invest more in it now, but neither of us regrets that choice. We try to be as honest with each other as we are with ourselves. We talk openly about our fears and our needs. If one of us has been unable to sleep, we share our worries the next day.

In many ways it is more difficult to watch the person you love suffer than to suffer yourself. I know that even when I sleep soundly at night, Les often wakes up in the wee hours and worries.

April 30, 1993

131

September 23, 1992
It was a beautiful fall day. We had lunch on the patio.

It has been more than three years since the CFS began and over two years since I was diagnosed with breast cancer.

I am grateful for the good days, which I treasure. I refuse to let the bad days get the better of me.

I am grateful for my family and friends who have lifted me up so many times, surrounded me with so much love, and shown so much patience with my limitations.

Notwithstanding, life is more a do-it-yourself job than one might imagine.

When She Is Four

My youngest granddaughter,
overjoyed to be visiting,
begged to take her morning bath
with me.

I said, "Of course, my love,"
not remembering
she would confront, for the first time,
my scarred and barren chest—
and she would wonder.
She will know someday, of course,
that my misfortune
increases her risk
(and that of her mother).

She will have to watch and worry,
check herself, be checked—
(there was no breast cancer
in my family history—
there is in hers).
I bequeath
a sinister possibility
to her—

But she doesn't have
to know
when she is four.

I sneak a quick shower—
tears and water streaming down my face—
and bathe her later.

September 1992

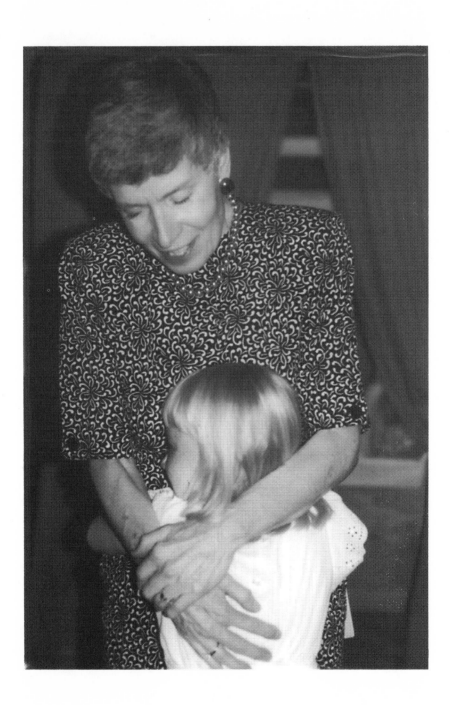

I Cannot Go with You All the Way

Connection

(for my beloved grandchildren)

I watch you playing on the beach
I run with you on the sand
I see you grow taller

I hear you speak with the wisdom of childhood
I find your eyes alight with understanding
I sense the integrity growing in your soul

You are
                my hope of immortality
                my extension of creativity
                my legacy of love

Together we walk toward tomorrow...

I cannot go with you all the way
But for now I hold your hand

And when I step aside

You, my precious one,
You will go on alone...

May 1992

And When She Was Bad

You've seen the ugly side of me
The livid, darkened, screwed up face
You've heard me shout some bitter words
(Intense for even human race)

You've watched me tear up tender roots
Of love, and hurl them to the wind
(In total rage at faith and light)
And wondered how some day I'd mend
The fences that are trampled down

And yet—your arms are always there
Your heart absorbs the fiercest blows
Your rough hands stroke my rumpled hair

You rock me 'til my inner child
Has spent her fury and her fear
And when she smiles and reaches out
She finds that you, my love, are here

June 1992

October 2, 1992

Rosalie [my best friend] called long distance this morning to tell me she is having a breast biopsy next week.

When I visited her in March, she told me that she was concerned about a mass in one breast. I urged her to see a surgeon. She told me this morning that the surgeon had reassured her and asked her to return in six months. Now a new doctor has asked for a biopsy.

But she didn't tell me last spring what happened, and somehow I had allowed myself to forget the conversation. I was horrified to realize that we could both fall into so much denial.

Had she told me what the surgeon said (or had I remembered to ask), I would have insisted that she get another opinion immediately, followed by a biopsy.

> I knew two women who died from breast cancer who had lumps that didn't show up on mammograms, even though they could easily feel them. Their doctors had also told them not to worry.

> Six months later, the husband of one finally demanded she have a biopsy. She had since discovered a lump in her other breast, but the doctor wasn't going to biopsy it until she insisted. Both lumps were cancerous, and there was cancer in all 26 lymph nodes they removed.

> She seemed to regain some quality of life for about eighteen months, but four years later she died of widely metastasized cancer.

> The second woman tried to ignore the fact that her lump was growing, and when she simply followed her doctor's directive to return in four months, he was shocked that it had become so large.

After her mastectomy, she told me that her prognosis was good—they had found cancer in only one lymph node. But she died within a year.

If Rosalie does have cancer, I wonder whether her having shared my cancer experience so intimately with me will make it easier for her. Or harder. I must be careful to let her start at the beginning and discover her own path, just as each of us must.

God, I hope she doesn't have cancer.

November 10, 1992

In January, when I first decided to include some journal entries with the poetry, I went back to my diaries for 1990 and 1991 and typed the raw material onto several pages for reference. Then I condensed the entries into one concise, unemotional page to introduce the book and went on with the project.

A few days ago, when Peggy questioned me about the lack of detail and, more importantly, about the lack of feeling on that page, I dismissed the questions, thinking that I had always handled the situation well.

When she pushed me to expand the information, I was forced back to the raw data, absolutely shocked by how much my present perception of what I had experienced differed from what I had written in my journals.

As I reread those entries, I realized how similar I was to the women who join our support group hoping to learn how to deal with their newly diagnosed cancer. How arrogant of me to think they should be where I am *now*. How essential it is that each woman ultimately find her own way. How important it is that I tell my story as it really happened, not as time has softened it in my memory.

And yet, as some come with their terror, I see myself and others still shrinking from recalling our early horror, trying to convince ourselves we were different from them.

And when others come with a strong sense of denial and a most determined bravery, I feel great sadness—seeing the cloak of innocence they wrap so carefully around them, unaware how much it has already frayed.

December 27, 1992

Recently after reading my journal entry of October 1991 and the three poems I wrote then, Peggy urged me to more deeply probe my feelings about dying. When she pressed me to recall my first experience with death, I thought of my playmate, Alma Lou, who died when we were five.

And then, almost as an afterthought, I remembered the loss of my dog, Collie, when I was three. (When I look at pictures of myself at age three, my heart aches as I see my vulnerability.) All the years of searching had never freed that memory before.

Now suddenly I understood more clearly the specter of Darkness that has haunted me for so much of my life. I wrote "My Voice Swept Away on the Wind" [p. 6] in response to this memory, grateful again for the way in which insights are still unfolding.

> Until I was almost thirty, I was able to accept the tenets of my church and society without much questioning. But as I look back, it is difficult for me to distinguish what my church taught from the dominant value system in the U. S. in the 1950's. So much was implied.

> It was the *Donna Reed* story. If you stay at home and care for the children.... If you do the laundry on Monday and clean the bathrooms on Friday.... If you bake cookies and make gingerbread houses.... If you try to make each Christmas happier than the last....

> But it became more and more difficult for me, and I eventually realized the truth of *Ecclesiastes:*

>> The race is not always to the swift nor the battle to the strong...but time and chance happen to them all. (9:11)

> And I knew what I had suspected all along—I would have to search for myself.

I continue to find much sustenance in my lifelong faith and in the church I have attended for 47 years. My convictions are deeply held—but the answers are not easy anymore.

My quest continues. And I am beginning to understand—the more clearly I see The Final Dark, the more I sense a Final Light.

The Rose

Perception unfolds
like the endless petals
of
an Infinite Rose

Surely
the center is
Light

December 1992

On Dying

There are two things that
bother me

I can't take
my teddy bear with me

and

I don't know
if there will be one
where I am going

January 8, 1993

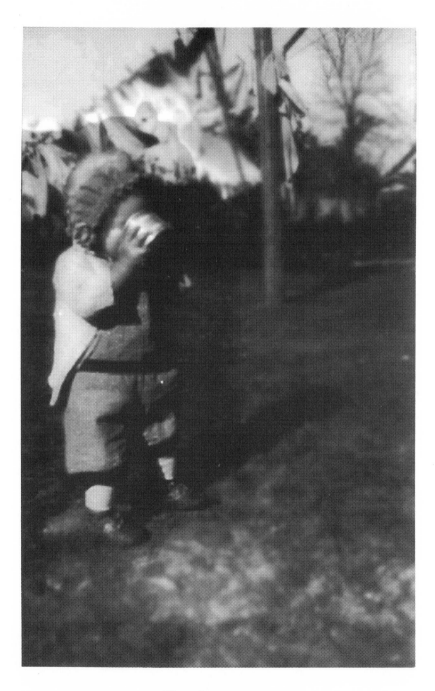

The author at age one.

As If It Were
the First Morning

January 21, 1993

Les brought daffodils from the grocery store today. He put them in a vase and set them on the kitchen table—harbingers of spring, symbols of sunshine.

I gaze at their freshness, reveling in the sense of renewal.

Blindsided

The internist was poker-faced.
"You know about this lump,
of course."

I returned his steady gaze.
"What lump?"

The surgeon was poker-faced.
"When do you want the biopsy?"

The kaleidoscope of my life
twisted into a nauseating pattern
of terrifying color
and jagged edges.

February 25, 1993

February 25, 1993

Les and I went to the clinic for our annual physicals this morning. All the lab tests were normal.

But when the doctor did the physical exam, he found several enlarged lymph nodes in my left armpit. He said he did not feel overly concerned, but he felt that I should check with my surgeon, which I was able to do right after lunch.

The surgeon said there are several possible reasons for such enlargements, but that the only way to rule out cancer would be to do a biopsy. Since the lumps are in such a sensitive place, I will need a general anesthetic. And I know that surgery always worsens my CFS.

It is all so unsettling to me. I don't understand how I failed to find the lumps myself. At least once a week, I poke and prod myself meticulously, searching for even the slightest grain of sand. I just did not dig deeply enough. It makes me wonder how I can monitor myself better.

I could ask Les to help me, but I know he would not be willing to hurt me by prodding deeply enough to find a lump. More importantly, I know his fingers would obey his heart, unwilling to find a lump that might contain the seed of my death.

I have realized once again that I do not have as much control over my destiny as I have imagined. But I do not think I could ever be as afraid as I was when they first diagnosed cancer.

Benign

benign, benign, benign
a benevolent word

how beneficial it is
to breathe again

March 1993

A Reflection on Worry

Each experience reveals how different people are. I think I was more afraid this week, after I *knew* the lumps were benign, than I was last week, when I knew I *might* have a recurrence of cancer. But the children and Les were more upset before the biopsy, and now they are relieved.

I mustered all my strength to get through the March piano recitals. I didn't want to squander any of my energy, thinking about the lumps the doctor had found in my armpit. I held up my guard through the surgery and over the weekend, while we awaited the official test results.

Then my guard dropped, and I began to think of the ramifications if the biopsy had revealed cancer. And I realized that *every* time I have a lump, they are going to have to take it out. They won't be able to wait and see, like they could with patients who have no history of cancer.

I had a lump removed from my jaw line in December 1991, only five months after my second mastectomy. It had not concerned me as much, perhaps because I had discovered it myself. And it was benign, just as the doctors had predicted. But these lumps worried me more—because I hadn't discovered them and because they were in my armpit—on the side where cancer had been confirmed. The doctors had again said they would be surprised to find cancer. But I told Les that if they were *really* sure the lumps were benign, they wouldn't have to take them out.

I did not tell anyone about this surgery except our children, my breast cancer support group, and Peggy. Each time I have had a biopsy or mastectomy (five surgeries in less than three years), I have struggled with whom to tell, when to tell, and how much to tell.

Each time the dilemma arises, I try to deal with it in a way that seems best for that event, balancing other people's changing needs with my own. I never feel that my decisions quite meet my needs or the needs of those close to me. I feel angry at having to be a public relations expert while I am dealing with so much else.

I would want to know about a test or an illness that my parents or my children had to face. I would want to know—no matter how much anxiety it caused me. I would feel blindsided if one of them were suddenly to announce, "The biopsy was malignant," if I hadn't even known there was a problem.

How differently I feel when I am the one facing cancer. Each time I have faced the possibility of cancer, I have wanted to keep it to myself—at least until I knew the results. My desire for privacy made it very difficult for Les when I had the first biopsy, in 1990. I was determined that no one else know I had cancer before I did. So he was placed in the tough position of having to be evasive with the children until he had told me—he simply told them that I had come through the surgery well. Eager to believe the best, they assumed he meant the biopsy was benign. But they were cruelly shocked when I called a few hours later to tell them that I had cancer.

My children tell me that they want to know the truth—including when I need to have a biopsy. They don't want to be blindsided any more than I do. On the other hand, my parents have said they don't want to know about tests until I have the results.

But I sense that sometimes my father finds it hard to believe I am telling him the entire truth about my health, even though I have never felt that he has doubted me otherwise. The week after my most recent biopsy, he and Les were on a church retreat. The first thing he asked Les when they were alone was how I *really* was. He told Les that he dreads the possibility that one of his children will die before he does.

Two days after the surgery, Les and I attended our church support group. Everyone was shocked, first by my wan appearance and then by my explanation. One friend commented, "I had just assumed that everything was fine with you—that you were beyond the worrying stage." The remark startled me. Recurrences of most cancers occur within the first few years, and it has been less than two years since my second mastectomy. But breast cancer can recur even twenty years later—I will *never* be past the worrying stage.

The members of the breast cancer support group are acutely aware of the risks. I could see the concern in their faces and sense their thinking "This could be me." People who have had cancer know the possibilities well: A malignant cell could survive to spread the cancer, or our healthy cells could turn on us again. Each time one of us confronts a new lump, each of us confronts the possibility of cancer in herself. There is no need to ask "for whom the bell tolls." And when the results are benign, it reassures us all.

Last night, there were two new women at the cancer support group. Arlene (a young mother) had a mastectomy last month and is facing chemotherapy. Carla had breast cancer in 1975. In 1987, she discovered that it had metastasized throughout her body. She has been in treatment with various hormone therapies ever since.

Arlene asked Carla, "How can you possibly deal with this day-to-day?" Carla simply said, "I've had a long time to get used to it, and I have a lot of treatment modes at my disposal. In three months, I'll get my nursing degree, and I'm very busy. You just can't think about it all the time."

I said, "After all, *life* is terminal....We simply live our lives as best we can."

After the meeting, I told Arlene that I used to worry about the remotest things that could happen to my children until my son, Russ, walked out of a vacation cabin when he was barely six. My daughter, Karen, had even blocked the door with her cot. But she had gotten up to go to the bathroom about midnight. Sleepwalking for the first time in his life, Russ pushed the aluminum cot aside and wandered into the night, miraculously surviving the dangers of that mountainous area and a creek for hours before the posse found him. I decided then that it was useless to worry—I could never have imagined the set of circumstances that allowed him to get out of that cabin unnoticed.

Although no one can avoid worry at some times, or even terror at others, I try to refrain from killing the time I have with dread of what *could* come to pass. I want to share the joy of living with those I love.

March 14, 1993

Shall We Dance?

Enter the Leper of Light!

See him smile and bow
See him pirouette
See his hand extended in
gracious invitation

See the people pale
and shrink away
wishing to dance with the Light
but
afraid of the Leper

See them huddle 'round the punch bowl
See them form a conga line
Listen to their idle chatter

Short-sighted creatures—
leprosy is only temporal

But if we fail to embrace the Light
we risk
dancing with Darkness
forever

1992

April 2, 1993

It was a long, hard winter. All the robins left this year. But now the grass is beginning to green and the daffodils are blooming.

I know the robins will come.

May 16, 1993

Today was truly special.

The church looked lovely for my students' big Spring Recital—the two pianos gleaming on the stage, the black-ink notes dancing on manuscript paper on the walls, and the sanctuary overflowing with baskets of red geraniums.

There were many more guests than I had expected; the students played well, and the joyful spirit which filled the room was almost palpable.

At the end of the program, I stood on my head. (For the past thirty years I did this on the last day of class for each group of students. The children always loved it. But this year, since I am not going to offer the bonus week of lessons after the recital, I decided to add another light touch to the program.)

I wasn't sure my arms would be strong enough to support my body today. Although I have stood on my head many times since the mastectomies, my practice head-stands two days ago weren't successful. But I decided to try anyway, and just to laugh if I failed. The important thing was to try.

Four years ago, I wouldn't have considered taking such a risk. But nothing seems much like a risk anymore. And my sense of decorum has yielded to my desire to find joy in everything I do.

I hadn't planned to make any closing remarks, but when I was preparing for the recital this morning, the following thoughts came to me and I decided to share them.

> It is to this time that I have come—
> to an afternoon such as this—
> full of music, children,
> laughter, learning, joy

It is to this time that I have come—
to claim my small space on the planet
to share what I can do
to stretch my talent
to take a risk

It is to this time that I have come—
but I couldn't be here without each of you
sharing, laughing, loving, encouraging

Thank you so much!

As we had refreshments, the children and their parents were beaming. Again and again, the children came up and hugged me to say goodbye for the summer.

As we embraced, I realized once more how much joy I find in teaching.

"And They All Lived Happily Ever After"

What is a happy ending?
How do I know that I'm happy?
When do I know I have ended?

May 25, 1993

A Reflection on Happy Endings

A few people who read drafts of this book felt that it is very sad and commented that they kept waiting for the happy ending. Their responses surprised me since others have said they felt uplifted and encouraged by the book.

Such opposite reactions made me think again about what constitutes a happy ending and—since many experiences don't end until we die—happiness in general.

I asked several friends, "What would you consider a happy ending?" One friend thought for a long time and then said, "If my husband and I could live a healthy, active life until age eighty and then die unexpectedly together."

Another friend, recently and suddenly widowed at the age of sixty, replied without any hesitation, "It would be to wake in the morning without the cold heaviness in my chest and to go to bed at night with peace of mind.... And I would like people to give me *time* to work through my grief."

Does a happy ending for cancer patients suggest that life must return to the way it was before cancer? Does a happy ending mean that there will never be any shadows? Does it imply that I must constantly wear a smile? Perhaps the issue is hard for me to deal with because I feel that having a smile deep in my heart—having come to terms with sorrow in life—is more important than wearing a smile on my face.

How can we tell if a person is happy? Some faces bubble over with joy, while the sadness in other faces seems to crush us. But it is impossible to tell whether most people are happy or sad simply by looking at them—a smile can mask great sorrow. I know I tend to be more reflective than a lot of people, but I do think of myself as a happy person.

It can be even more difficult to infer people's emotions from their writing. My writing seems so transparent to me that I wondered how anyone reading this book could have

158

missed the blossoms of joy and humor that have sustained me during the past four years—my relationship with Les, my teaching, and the blooming of the daffodils and the return of the robins after a long winter.... Perhaps I am too subtle. Perhaps I should stand on my head more often.

Sometimes I wish that life were less complicated—that joy was always unadulterated, that happiness was always untempered. But life consists of "and-ness." It is pleasure *and* pain, health *and* illness, joy *and* sorrow. If we miss a moment of joy while we are immersed in sorrow, we miss that particular joy forever. It is a question of savoring the roses even though we are aware of the thorns.

When I was first diagnosed with breast cancer, I bargained for just two more years of life (forgetting how short two years could be). I have had those two years and more. At this point my cancer prognosis is good although I still struggle with CFS.

Cancer has forced me to consider the issues of dying, and CFS has demanded that I search for solutions to living. These fine black lines on starchy white paper have been lifelines in my struggle.

In some ways my life has been distilled to its essence. It is easier now to concentrate on what is important to me—meeting my own expectations rather than others'; walking alone in fresh-fallen snow; taking a grandchild to McDonald's or the park; gathering my family or friends around a beautifully set table for a simple supper; decorating the house for Christmas; and, most of all, waking at night to gently touch Les's face and be grateful for our long years together.

As I listened to the students playing their own compositions [May 16], I remembered how uptight I used to get about the Spring Recital, worrying about all the details. Were the printed programs letter-perfect? Would the children forget their pieces? Could I play *my* piece flawlessly?

Everyone was together; everyone was watching. Would I live up to their expectations?

As I listened, I realized I have changed. Now I tell my students (and myself) that the walls will not cave in if we mis-play a few notes—the important thing is to create beauty and joy, to give it our best and to have fun while we are doing it.

Perhaps it is only when we truly understand that our lives will not be perfect that we have the freedom to venture into the rose garden without worrying about scratches from the thorns.

I believe that it is possible to find some joy in almost every experience.

A conversation with my recently widowed friend confirmed that belief. In spite of her deep grief, she treasures the kindnesses that are gracing her life—a poem from a fifth grader where she teaches, the gift of a friendly schnauzer to keep her company, a long letter of condolence from an old friend, the incredible feeling of being enveloped in the love of friends near and far.

What *is* a happy ending? Is it having a face without wrinkles? Is it never being ill or disappointed? Is it never losing a loved one? I think not—because if a happy ending is those things, most of us are going to miss it.

For me, a happy ending is the knowledge that, even though the flame may flicker, my inner candle of joy burns brightly.

I have found an immense awareness, an incredible joy in treasuring each moment—and a profound gratitude that greets each new dawn as if it were the First Morning.

May 17, 1993
June 4, 1993

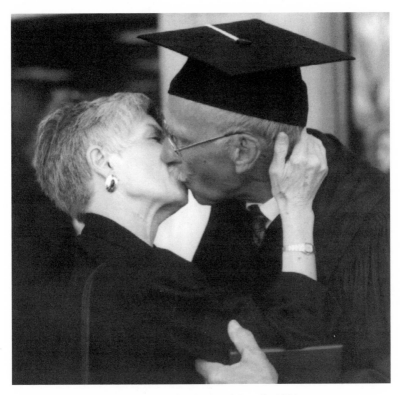

The author and her husband, Les, in 1991.

Index

Poems

Titled Prose

Fine Black Lines is available through your local bookstore or directly from the publisher:

> Mulberry Hill Press
> Box 425 B
> Englewood, CO 80151
> (1-800-294-4714)

Book *Fine Black Lines* $14.95

Shipping Regular Mail—first book 2.50
Each additional book .75
Priority Mail—first book 3.50
Each additional book 1.00

Sales Tax Colorado (in Denver) add 1.10
Colorado (outside Denver) add .45

To Order Send name, address, and MC/Visa number with expiration date or check payable to Mulberry Hill Press. Phone orders accepted at 1-800-294-4714.

If you are interested in having the author read or speak to a group, contact Mulberry Hill Press.